HAIRSTYLING

AT

HOME

To Linda
who is always an inspiration

To Lisa and Gina
who cut each other's hair at the ages
of four and five and thought we wouldn't notice

HAIRSTYLING

AT

HOME

by

Richard Gilroy

Illustrated by Jane Pirie

PAPERFRONTS

ELLIOT RIGHT WAY BOOKS

KINGSWOOD, SURREY, U.K.

Typeset in 10pt Times by One & A Half Graphics, Redhill, Surrey.
Made and Printed in Great Britain by Cox & Wyman Ltd., Reading, Berkshire.

CONTENTS

PREFACE

I have spent the last fifteen years hairdressing, and building a business with my wife who is also a qualified hairstylist. Together we continue to learn and teach our staff within our two salons.

A good teacher never stops learning and is always on the look out for new ideas, new ways of cutting and styling hair. As an apprentice, I used to take the best from every hairstylist that I came in contact with, finding that they all had their strengths and weaknesses. This way I learned many different methods of hairstyling. Together my wife and I have attended numerous hairdressing courses in the hope of finding some new rare gem of knowledge.

The purpose of this book is to give you all the basic information you need in order to look after a person's hair. It also contains useful tips and hints on keeping your hair looking good between visits to your regular hairstylist, as well as a section aimed at helping anyone interested in becoming a hairdresser or setting up in business.

INTRODUCTION

Over the last few years the term barber has begun to die out and be replaced by hairdresser, hairstylist, unisex hairstylist, and hair artist. Of course some barber shops can still be found, and even some modern salons have been called barber shops in the desire to be different and win trade, but this is generally thought unfashionable nowadays.

The term *barber* is derived from the Latin word *barbe* which loosely means beard. Hairdressers have been around since the dawn of mankind in one form or another. Many modern styles can be traced back to ancient civilisations, such as the square bob which is very much like the ancient Egyptian style. The Egyptians even had their own method of perming hair.

Many years ago, barbers did some of the tasks of surgeons! When bleeding was considered the right way to combat some illnesses, the barber's pole was said to represent a pole used during bleeding. Bandages were wrapped around the pole and it was placed outside the shop to indicate the presence of a barber-surgeon.

Eventually the true meaning of the pole disappeared and it simply became a trademark of the barber's shop.

Many of the methods of hairdressing have improved over the centuries but some seemingly modern methods aren't too different from the techniques used in the days of yore.

One famous name in hairdressing is Marcel Grateau who invented the Marcel waving iron in 1872-73. These irons were of various sizes, and they were placed in stoves to heat up before they were used to curl hair. Modern-day tongs are still very similar to the marcel irons and the methods he used to create waves and curls were similar to the ones used today.

The skills involved in hairdressing are many; the techniques used in many modern salons may differ greatly, but hairdressing remains an art. Just as artists have different styles of painting, so hairdressers may use a variety of methods to achieve the same end result. Learning the many skills can be fun as well as rewarding; many of the old barbers' methods still exist and as long as the more adventurous hairdressers search for new methods of styling hair and re-discover the old ways, they will never die. Anyone can learn hairdressing, and with practice a reasonable level of skill can be acquired.

GLOSSARY

ALOPECIA — Hair loss.

ANAGEN — Stage where hair growth is most active.

BOB — A one length style that has many variations.

BODY — The thickness and volume of hair.

CALFLICK — See 'Widow's peak'.

CATAGEN — Stage of hair growth where growth stops.

COMBING IN — Combing the hair into a nice style after it has been blow-dried or set.

CORTEX — Part of hair that contains disulphide linkages.

CRIMPING-IRON — Heating iron used to produce pattern in hair.

CROWN — Whirl of hair at the top of the head that denotes the hair's natural movement.

CUTICLE — Outer layer of hair, consisting of scales.

CUTS, DIFFERENT TYPES OF	See page 31.
DISULPHIDE LINKAGES	Bonds in hair that form its shape.
DOUBLE CROWN	A whirl of hair at each side of the top of the head.
FOLLICLE	Depression in skin from which hair grows.
HYDROGEN PEROXIDE	Oxidising agent used in hairdressing.
KERATIN	Hard protein which makes up most of human hair.
LANUGO HAIR	Downy hair; baby hair.
MEDULLA	The inner core of the hair.
MELANIN	Pigment that gives hair darker colour.
MOVEMENT	The hair's *natural* movement is the direction it will fall without any styling. However, we can *add* movement to hair (i.e. make the hairs within a hairstyle move in contrasting directions) by giving the hair curls and waves.
PAPILLA	Part of hair from which hair shaft grows.
PERIMETER	The edge, or base line, of the hairstyle that forms its outer shape – its contour.

PHEOMELANIN	Pigment which forms light colours.
PIN TAIL COMB	The same as a tail comb but with a metal tail (see fig. 16).
PSORIASIS	Non-contagious skin disease similar to dandruff but more severe.
SEBACEOUS GLANDS	Glands which produce sebum.
SEBUM	The hair's natural oils.
SECTIONS	In the process of cutting, perming, colouring and styling hair, strands of hair are gathered together into sections away from the rest of the hair. If cutting hair, each section should be about ¼ inch thick, and if blow-waving, about ½ inch thick. With cutting, once the first section is cut to the required length, that section is used as a guide for the remaining sections. This ensures an accurate cut. When drying hair, it is divided into sections so that each part of the hair is styled and dried correctly before moving on to the next section. This helps to avoid mistakes.
STYLES, DIFFERENT	See page 40.
TAIL COMB	The same as a pin tail comb but with a plastic tail (see fig. 16).
TELOGEN	Resting stage of hair growth.
TRICHOSIDERIN	Pigment that produces reddish shades.

VOLUME   The amount of hair on the head.

WIDOW'S PEAK   Hair at the front hairline that
                         shoots away from the rest of the
                         hair's natural movement. Some-
                         times known as a 'calflick'.

1

ALL ABOUT HAIR

Hairdressing jargon

It may help if I explain at the outset some of the technical terms used by hairdressers. I have often heard clients asking questions of young stylists and seen them bewildered by the words used to describe such things as the stages of hair growth, or the techniques of perming hair.

On average, those of us not suffering from hair loss have somewhere in the region of 100,000 hairs on our heads, give or take a few thousand. A strand of hair starts growing from the papilla, which is rather like a bud. If a hair is plucked out, usually the growing process will simply start again. The root is enclosed by the hair follicle, and a hair is thickest at its root. If the hair is cut, the hair does not grow any thicker, but because the hair is thicker at the root and middle length this appears to be the case.

A hair has three layers. The outermost layer is called the cuticle, which consists of scales that protect the hair. These are arranged rather like the tiles on a roof. The next layer is called the cortex. This allows the hair to be stretched and holds pigment which provides the colour. The middle part is called the medulla. This is soft and spongy and is sometimes absent in fine hair; generally it is in proportion as the lead in a pencil.

Hair reflects our state of health. It is fed by the blood, and therefore is affected by diet as well as by medication, etc. Hair is mainly protein, therefore protein is needed in the diet to keep it healthy. Generally a healthy diet is also the correct diet for a good head of hair.

Hair is not living tissue; it is dead from the point where it comes out from the body, but it may continue to grow for up to as many as six years. Wearing your hair is similar to wearing a woolly jumper or the skin of animals which we call leather. Leather or wool and human hair can all be kept in beautiful condition.

The majority of us lose about one hundred hairs per day. They fall out but are usually replaced, so there is no cause for worry.

The hair is protected by natural oils, but split ends occur easily because the natural oils do not reach the ends of long hair to protect it. Therefore when growing hair, it is wise to have the split ends cut every six weeks. If the split ends are left unattended they will spread up the hair shaft, and then the only cure is to cut them off.

The protein that makes up most of the hair is called *keratin*, which is composed of amino acids. Hair is made up of the elements of nitrogen, phosphorus, carbon, hydrogen, sulphur, and chlorine.

Hair contains pigment which supplies colour: Melanin (brown-black); Pheomelanin (brownish-yellow), etc.

A mixture of these different types of pigment supplies the contrasting shades apparent on some heads of hair.

When the body is beginning to run down through age or illness, it can no longer create hair pigment, and this is when the hair begins to go grey.

Hair can be stretched and will jump back to its original length unless it has been damaged. This allows us to set, or blow-wave hair. Hair is stretched and wound round the roller and then dried. It will hold its roll until water allows it to jump back to its original shape. This is what gives hair its strength, and is the source of the story of the maiden who lets down her hair to be used as rope in order to be rescued.

Stages of growth

Hair has three main stages of growth: Telogen, Anagen A and B, and Catagen.

TELOGEN

A state of rest where no growth occurs. If this state continues indefinitely, alopecia (baldness) may occur.

ANAGEN A

The hair starts to grow. Sometimes it remains undeveloped and lanugo hair develops. This is a soft sort of weak hair. Sometimes hair tonics help to produce this effect, but the hair falls out easily and the tonics must be used frequently to maintain the effect. This is the type of hair babies have when they are born.

ANAGEN B

The hair grows properly for anything up to six years; the length of your hair depends on how long the Anagen B stage lasts.

CATAGEN

The hair falls out, the papilla goes back into the rest state (Telogen stage).

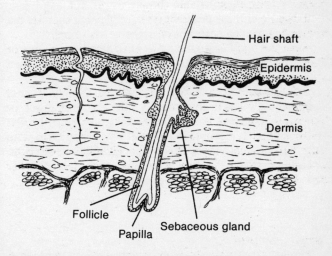

Fig. 1. The root of the hair.

Fig. 1 gives an idea of the way hair grows, showing the sebaceous gland that surrounds the hair root and the papilla. Hair is in some respects like a plant growing in a garden; it draws nourishment from the blood stream in order to grow into a healthy-looking hair.

The angle of hair growth

Fig. 2 will give you an idea of the natural direction of hair growth and the type of cutting angle that may be necessary. Apart from the crown, or widow's peaks (calflicks) and whirls in the hair, all hair follows this direction of growth. The angle of growth is rather like the direction of spokes on a bicycle wheel from its centre. Very strong hair sticks out at this angle showing off the hair's movement (see the glossary) and giving the spiked effect.

Here you can see how the cutting line could easily be altered to shape hair in more, or feather the fringe, etc.

Most layer cutting is done in such a way as to follow this natural movement.

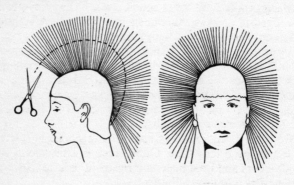

Fig. 2.   The hair's natural angle of growth.

What makes hair shiny?

The cuticle consists of overlapping scales; when the hair is wet they are open, and when dry they close. When they lie smoothly, they reflect light and give hair its shine. When they become damaged, the hair becomes dull.

Conditioning works by closing all the cuticle scales, thus making the hair shine. Conditioners only affect the outer layer of hair and concentrate on smoothing the cuticle scales down. Some colours, such as blonde shades, give the appearance of shining more as well, because they reflect more of the colour spectrum.

Straightening curly or wavy hair

The methods employed for straightening hair in my opinion are not very effective. In our salons we usually try to talk people out of having their hair straightened. One method employs practically the same principles as for perming hair, but flattens the hair and drags it straight. Usually the hair doesn't straighten completely and often loses its condition, weakening it and leaving it dry and split. I prefer to offer a selection of alternative hairstyles rather than to try to straighten the hair.

Hair problems – how to cope

Many people suffer from conditions such as greasy or dry hair, dandruff, flyaway unmanageable hair, etc. All of these problems can be treated with the right product.

Sometimes the significance of hair problems is exaggerated especially in advertisements. Often they are just natural phases the body goes through. Hair treatments are necessary only when problems become severe. Extreme scalp disorders or nervous problems should be referred to your local doctor or specialist.

When using hair products, some treatments should usually be left on for a long time. Often, even in hair salons, hair conditioners and treatments are rinsed off before they have had a chance to take full effect.

When applying a hair treatment or tonic at home, comb it in thoroughly and then cover the hair with a plastic bag. This helps the product to soak right through into the hair. Leave it on for as long as half-an-hour if it is just an ordinary conditioner and the instructions don't state otherwise. The hair cuticle will be smoothed down leaving each hair shiny and manageable.

HAIR LOSS

For men suffering from loss of hair, my advice is to keep the style short. Don't try to compensate by growing the hair you have, in order to conceal the hair loss, because it usually looks unnatural. Putting low partings in the hair to sweep what remaining hair there is across the head will only draw attention to the problem. Many famous people cope with the difficulty admirably, indeed some of them are even known as sex symbols and they make no effort to hide their baldness.

GOING GREY

For those who are going grey, I do recommend colouring hair, but the colour needs to look natural. By staying close to your natural colour it won't be so apparent that your hair has been coloured.

If you want to colour your own hair, don't go out and buy the first colour that takes your fancy. There are many makes on the market, some good, some bad.

Consider having it coloured by a professional. A good hairstylist can play around with colour, creating the best shade for you. There is a right way to apply colour to hair, and the hairdresser has the experience.

DISASTERS

Unfortunately, bad judgment (sometimes even by the hairstylist) may result in catastrophe. It may be a perm or highlights, or even a haircut. Often the best thing to do, if possible, is to leave well alone. If it is a perm, it may go from bad to worse when permed again.

The problem may have begun at the very start, the hairstylist may not have understood the required style. Sometimes it may be just lack of experience. In any job there are good and bad tradesmen.

Find another hairdresser, talk over the problem. Sometimes a bad haircut can be altered or, if your hair is in good condition, a re-perm may work. It may be that the first hairdresser wasn't to blame for the mistake. There are many possible reasons for a bad result: ill health, medication, faulty products are just some.

PSORIASIS

This is a skin disease which could affect any part of the body. When it attacks the scalp it often looks like a harsh form of dandruff. It is best referred to your doctor as the disease is a chronic one and difficult to clear up.

DRY HAIR

Dry hair can be caused by a number of things. Incorrect use of certain hair treatments. Sunlight drying hair out too much. Lack of sebum (natural oils) coming from sebaceous glands. Sebaceous glands can be stimulated with correct shampooing which massages the scalp whilst washing the hair. Plenty of conditioner should put the hair back into a healthy-looking state.

INFECTIONS AND SCALP PROBLEMS

Infections and other scalp conditions should be taken into consideration before styling hair. Here are a few of the problems that may be found.

RINGWORM is a fungal type of infection. It can cause the hair to fall out if severe. Contrary to what the name suggests, there is no worm involved. Ringworm can lead to an even worse fungal infection called favus. The skin goes yellow and dry and flaky. As soon as ringworm appears, ask your doctor for advice.

BOILS are a nasty type of infection. If they are swollen and on the verge of bursting or have burst, then no hair chemicals such as perm lotions, etc., should be used until the problem clears up.

This also applies to moles, warts, cuts and wounds, or open sores of any kind.

CYSTS are sometimes found on the scalp. They are caused if a sebaceous gland becomes blocked. The gland's job is to produce oil, and a build up of oil creates a lump. Cysts can grow quite large. If they burst or become infected, obviously again no hair chemicals should be used.

HEAD LICE. One of the most embarrassing problems, especially for children, is head lice. They may catch them at school or even playing outside with other children. There's no need to panic, most chemists sell treatments that will remove them with a couple of applications.

It should also be remembered that, when cutting hair, hairdressers may pass on infections, perhaps from warts or from open sores on the hands.

All infections should be referred to your doctor.

SPLIT ENDS

Sadly, the only way to get rid of split ends is to cut them off before they spread down the hair shaft. With long hair, even if you're trying to grow it, have the split ends cut off every six weeks. Some hair-brushes can damage your hair. If your hair is splitting and becoming very brittle, then be especially gentle when shampooing and conditioning, and be particularly careful with tools.

PONY TAILS

I often see children in the salon with tight elastic bands around their hair to keep a pony tail in. Elastic bands are very bad for hair. They are too rough and they can cause hair damage. I would suggest the use of ribbon or a soft cord or even wool.

SUDDEN CHANGE OF CONDITION

Severe problems can sometimes be caused by worry and stress, or even a serious shock. The old story of someone's hair going grey because of a fright is not far from the truth. Obviously the ultimate solution is to search for a healthier and less worrisome lifestyle. All sorts of hair problems can be caused by stress, even harsh forms of dandruff or greasy hair. A change in hair condition may also come about through a change in diet or perhaps medication.

Hair changes condition as we grow older. It usually becomes dry and less shiny, and begins to lose its colour.

HAIR PROBLEMS DURING PREGNANCY

Usually any problems that occur during pregnancy will clear up when baby is born and your hair will revert to normal. You may even suffer hair loss, but it should correct itself in most cases. Unless the problem is really extreme, don't worry about it. Your hair may become greasy, or dry, or oddly enough, it may even seem to be in better condition than usual.

If you don't want to spend a lot of time on your hair during pregnancy and you want a new hairstyle, I advise a short layered style – perhaps feathery around the face. This is easy to look after and always looks neat with minimum fuss.

WIDOW'S PEAKS, DOUBLE CROWNS, WHIRLS, BALD PATCHES, AND OTHER NUISANCES

These usually can't be removed permanently, but there are one or two tricks that can make the hair look smart regardless. One method of hiding a widow's peak is to cut the fringe at a slight angle. When the fringe jumps up at the widow's peak it ends up looking straight. In reality the hair at the widow's peak is slightly longer, but it doesn't show. A rule to follow with hair of this kind is: don't fight it; follow its natural movement. When drying hair, blowing against the movement will only make it stick up more.

Gone are the days of boys' partings on the left and girls' on the right. You can make a widow's peak or double crown look right by using its strong movement to form the parting on whichever side suits.

The hair may have a whirl which is similar to a crown – again, it is often because it has been combed against its natural movement. Sometimes hair will even fall naturally into a parting from the widow's peak. You can find your natural parting, if you have one, by wetting your hair down and combing it back from your brow to your crown. This always works better when the hair is wet. Then follow the rule of not fighting the natural movement and avoid all sorts of difficulties. In some cases, the hair will not fall into a parting in this way, but that's no problem. Simply wet the hair down, comb it forward and then choose the necessary comb track for your parting.

There are occasions when a small bald patch may be covered by growing the hair slightly longer in that place. This usually only looks right when the problem is minor.

GREASY HAIR

The causes of greasy hair can be many: ill health, medication, too much fatty food, etc.

There are a couple of things to remember about washing greasy hair. A rough scrubbing action may seem to be the answer, but this will only stimulate the sebaceous glands, making the problem worse. Gentle action is all that is needed. Vary the types of shampoo you use. A shampoo specifically recommended for greasy hair should stop the greasiness, but when used frequently it will also remove the hair's natural oils and make it dry. Therefore only use the anti-grease shampoo until the condition improves. Then, a normal shampoo can be used instead. If you leave conditioner on your hair after shampooing this will also make the hair greasy, so rinse thoroughly.

Greasy hair is often caused by diet – too much fatty food – so usually healthy living means healthy hair.

FINE HAIR

This type of hair is delicate and should be treated carefully. Be cautious with perms, colours, or lighteners. Most hair lightening, bleaching and highlighting is done with hydrogen peroxide. When this is used incorrectly, it can burn and severely damage the hair.

Fine hair can be made to look thicker with short layer cuts. Hair is actually thicker at the roots and thinner at the ends. Keeping fine hair long may make the problem worse. Hair tends to fall out more easily when it is long.

DANDRUFF

Dandruff is unsightly and there are many products on the market to combat it, most of which contain virtually the same chemicals. Sometimes anti-dandruff treatments make the hair very dry and the dandruff just comes back a few days later. Everyone has dandruff in varying degrees. Ordinary dandruff is natural. We simply shed our old skin. I agree that it looks nasty, but the television commercials would have us believe it's some kind of disease.

THINGS THAT MAY DAMAGE YOUR HAIR

The list of things that may damage your hair is long; here are some to avoid.

If you like sunbathing when on holiday, remember to protect your hair as well as your body. The sun can do a lot of damage but this can be avoided easily by putting plenty of conditioner on your hair. This will work just as effectively as the expensive special products designed to protect your hair while sunbathing. The conditioner provides a protective coating which covers the cuticle and prevents heat damage.

A problem caused by swimming at the public baths can also be avoided with the use of conditioner. The chlorine in the water leaves hair dry and brittle. Always condition your hair after a swim; rinse all the chlorine out thoroughly.

Even the tools we use to style hair can do serious damage if used incorrectly. When blowing hair dry with a hairdryer, remember to keep the dryer moving. Keep it a couple of inches away from the scalp to avoid burning and singeing. Be careful not to get hair tangled in the back of the hairdryer.

When combing and brushing hair do not brush towards the root. This will cause the cuticle to break, causing loss of shine and split ends. Brushing hair the correct way helps to create a nice shine. When using tongs, don't hold hair in them for too long. A good method of avoiding damage is to put hair around the tongs and count 'one, two, three', then tong the next piece of hair similarly. This avoids causing any split ends.

Most hair products require a certain amount of professional skill to be applied correctly. If you have to apply them yourself, read the instructions carefully and find out what they contain. Remember with things other than basic conditioners we are often dealing with powerful chemicals that can do a lot of harm when wrongly used. Even when properly supervised I would advise a rest period for the hair between perms and colours or highlights. If your hair is in good condition, give it a two to three month gap between perms. If the hair is in very poor condition, give it a longer rest period. The same applies to highlights. Highlighting your hair too frequently will make it more blonde each time. You would lose the colour contrast created by the first highlighting.

If your hair is very dry, then having it permed or highlighted will only make the condition worse.

When you are ill you will find your hair suffers because hair mirrors health. It may go lank, losing its natural shine, or it may go very greasy. Condition your hair more than usual and perhaps try a new style to brighten you up.

Certain hard-bristle brushes and metal combs are much too hard on the hair and scalp. Many good hairstylists would throw some tools into the bin as they simply ruin hair. The metal comb comes in handy for combing hair into style when it has become static but is not for general use. Beware of tools with sharp pointed teeth and harsh bristles.

Hair tonics

"Doctor, my hair's falling out in clumps, have you got anything to keep it in?"

The doctor hands the gentleman a box.

Although this is rather a cruel joke, it's not far from the truth. There is a saying in the hairdressing world: "If you find the cure for baldness you'll soon be a millionaire." Many firms claim that their tonics cure baldness, but most of them, at the very best, give the effect of thickening hair. I am sure that scientists will come up with a permanent cure for baldness eventually, but meanwhile there are some excellent toupees, and hair transplants are also becoming increasingly popular.

Hair conditioners and treatments for greasy or dry hair certainly work, but many hair restorers and miracle cures for baldness are merely ways of taking money under false pretences.

Nature is full of things that are good for hair condition. Hairdressers have been known to make up their own hair tonics from the strangest things, such as beer, fruit, eggs, milk, coconuts, nettles and many more. Hair tonics can give hair a healthy shine, remove grease, add body, etc.

In a salon where I worked as an apprentice, one hairdresser used to make a hair tonic out of a mixture of eggs and milk.

GOOD THINGS FOR HAIR STRAIGHT FROM THE KITCHEN CUPBOARD

Most manufactured products contain natural ingredients in some form. All of the following things can be used for rinses, treatments, and shampoos. Many of them are just as good, if not better, than the manufactured products. Some of the ingredients may need liquidising before use. Experiment with them; mix different ingredients together. Leave them on your hair for about fifteen minutes. This is only a small selection. There are many more.

Apples, oranges, lemons, limes, melons, cherries, avocados, pineapples, tomato juice, beer, cider, wine, vinegar, eggs, milk, cucumber, honey, rosewater, yoghurt, mayonnaise, oatmeal, herbs, oris root, arrow root, sunflower oil, castor-oil, vegetable oil, almond oil, olive oil, wheatgerm oil, sesame oil, avocado oil.

All kinds of things have been used in the past to enrich the quality of human hair. Many have been supposedly "magic" formulae to make hair grow again. Every country has had its share of amazing potions to cure baldness, sold by merchants, door-to-door salesmen, and even so-called "hair specialists".

Romany gypsies (said to originate from the ancient Egyptians) made a living selling such magic potions and charms. Their Chovahanis "witches" would know all sorts of secret mixtures made from herbs and fruit. Some of them were hair potions, some of them health potions. Things beneficial to hair can be found literally everywhere. Seaweed, cactus plants, even blood in olden times was used as a colourant for hair.

Useful tips

Finding a good hairstylist can be difficult. As with other trades, the best do not always work at the largest salons. A good hairstylist will have undergone proper professional training. You will usually find that a good hairdresser spends a lot of time talking about your hair. This way mistakes are avoided. There will be many styles that suit you, but if you just leave everything up to the hairdresser, you may leave the salon with a style you hate. The good hairdresser will offer you a choice of styles. Be sure your mind is made up before proceeding with the cut.

There may be special tools sold in shops specifically for cutting your own hair. Most of these employ a thinning blade and without special supervison they will merely shred your hair. To cut your own hair properly you would literally need eyes in the back of your head.

The general opinion in the trade is to have your hair cut every six weeks on average. Some people have very fast growing hair and some slow. Some hairstyles lose their shape quickly and in these cases, if you can afford it, a more regular visit to the salon may be necessary.

2

CHOOSING THE STYLE AND GETTING PREPARED

Types of hair

EUROPEAN HAIR
 On the whole it is finer than Asian hair and varies widely in colour.

ASIAN HAIR
 Hair is usually dark and coarser and straight.

NEGROID HAIR
 Hair is usually curly and dark. When cut properly, some beautiful style shapes can be achieved from it. The curly perm or afro styles achieve the same effect.

 It's pleasing to see that, though each race has its own hair type, styles are admired and copied in the salon. Because of this, hairdressing helps break down some of the barriers between different cultures.
 Every hair type is plagued with the same hair problems and possesses fine hair, thick hair, dry hair, greasy hair, etc.
 Each hair type must be handled and cut and styled in an appropriate way. For example, really thick coarse hair must be divided into very fine sections before cutting, otherwise scissor marks will be visible at the end of the cut. The afro style has its own particular haircutting method which is overlooked at many hairdressing schools and requires a great

deal of practice. It relies on creating a perfect contour. You draw the hair out with the afro comb and actually cut a contour with the scissors or clippers.

The strange thing I have found in my hairdressing career is the high proportion of people who want the opposite hair type to the one they have got. Often, the person admired for beautiful curly hair wants straight hair, or the blonde wants dark hair, or perhaps in men the ability to grow a thick dark beard. Or the redhead wants to be a blonde.

This makes the job more interesting. The challenge for me is to make someone look completely different, and, if possible, more attractive, with a new hairstyle.

Methods of cutting

CLIPPER CUTTING

Clippers are an essential and sometimes underrated hairdressing tool. On first impressions clipper cutting looks easy, but some very clever styling can be carried out with clippers, which is more of a skilled job.

POINT CUTTING

This is a scissor cutting method, using only the points of the scissors to thin the hair.

RAZOR CUTTING

Razor cutting can produce some attractive styles when in the right hands, but I have seen some hairstyles ruined by incorrect use of the razor. It can also be used to thin hair out. The razor is only used on wet hair. Razor cutting is a skilful art; most of the movement comes from the wrists.

SLITHER CUTTING

A method of thinning hair by slithering the scissors down the hair shaft.

THINNING SCISSORS

These scissors have gained a bad reputation in recent years, but only because of improper use. When used properly, they can feather hair and remove scissor marks from a badly done layer cut. They have a serrated edge and can be used to thin out the last half inch of thick hair when doing a normal layer cut. If used wrongly, they easily make a mess of the hairstyle.

Types of cut

ASYMMETRIC CUTS

These styles are cut to different lengths at each side. They may even be cut in completely different ways, mixing up methods of cutting, perhaps cut very short at one side and graduated, but left one length at the other side and very long.

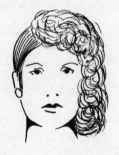   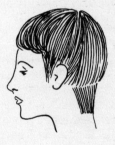

Fig. 3. Asymmetric cut.   **Fig. 4.** Cap.

CAP

The cap has many uses, it looks like a hat from the back when cut well. Styles like this have been known as the French beret or even the mushroom effect.

D/A NECKLINE

Hair at the rear of the head is combed into the middle from each side. The finished result resembles the pattern of a duck's backside.

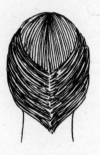

Fig. 5. D/A neckline.

FEATHERED CUT

This method is used to give a soft wispy finish at the fringe, or all over. It is created by using scissors or a razor. It can even be done with thinning scissors when used properly. Hair is cut at varying lengths instead of straight to create feathery styles or a style such as that sometimes known as the shake.

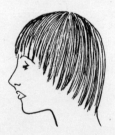

Fig. 6. Feathered cut.

FLAT TOP
    This is a spiked hairstyle, cropped very close at the sides and back, and cut short and square on the top so that it sticks up and is perfectly flat on top.

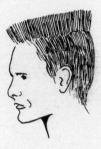

Fig. 7. Flat top.

GRADUATION
    Has many meanings but perhaps the most common is cutting the perimeter (or base line) of long hairstyles, such as bobs, etc., into long layers that usually go from short to longer at the edge. Graduation is done in stages of length. It can be used to create movement in the hair for styles like wedges, etc.

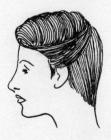

Fig. 8. Graduated style.

LAYERED OR CLUB CUTTING

Hair is cut to the same length all over. The layer cut is the most versatile of haircuts. There are many variations of layer cut and countless layer cut styles. Layer cutting should be done on wet hair for best results and is ideal for both men and women.

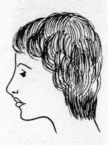

Fig. 9.   Layered or club cut.

ONE LENGTH

No layers, hair is cut along the perimeter in a number of styles such as pageboys and bobs, etc.

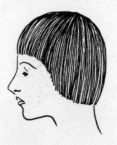

Fig. 10   One length.

PAGEBOY

A pageboy is a long bob that has a diagonal edge from the fringe to the bottom of the ears to the nape.

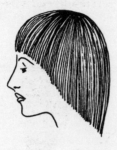

Fig. 11.   Pageboy.

SHINGLE

The shingle has many variations but it is a term not used very much now. Shingling is another form of graduation used to shape styles into the nape. The cut follows the contour of the neckline and is shaped in very short at the lower part of the nape.

Some hairdressers favour dry cutting for shingling and tapering, it is purely a matter of opinion and skill.

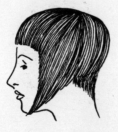

Fig. 12.   Shingle.

SPIKY

Spiky is a general term for most styles, even 'punk' styles, that stick up away from the head. As the name implies, the hair is cut short enough to spike. Some variation of a spike is always in fashion. The spike usually works better with strong hair that will stand up from the scalp, but gels and fixing sprays can be used with fine hair.

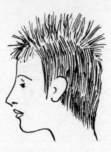

Fig. 13. Spiky.

SYMMETRIC CUTS

These styles are of even proportion with both sides balanced and cut to the same length. Sometimes styles look symmetrical but in reality they are not, because a lot of people have slightly asymmetrical features such as one ear lower than the other.

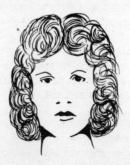

Fig. 14. Symmetric cut.

TAPER

This has a similar meaning to graduation. The expression is often used for very short styles, where it means that the hair is longer at the top of the head, and gets shorter as it goes towards the nape, eventually tapering away into nothing. The base line (or perimeter) vanishes completely.

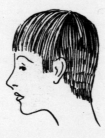

Fig. 15. Taper.

There are many other types of cut, such as concave and convex, which speak for themselves. New ideas are being created all the time. This is one of the things that make hairdressing exciting – a stylist can invent a completely new hairstyle.

In many haircuts, the different methods of cutting are mixed together to create the finished style. Several different types of cutting and hairdressing tools may be used for one haircut. In some salons only a limited range of methods is used. I find it best to employ as many methods as possible – sometimes a unique finish can be produced by using a cutting method that is even a little dated.

HOW YOUNG STYLISTS LEARN

Learning to cut hair well needs lots of patience and plenty of practice. When youngsters start working for us we give them certain things to practise, such as how to hold a pair of scissors properly. Hairdressers hold scissors with the third

finger and thumb for better balance and grip. This takes time
to get used to. We demonstrate the pattern needed for the first
basic cut, and then we sit someone down and let the learner
go through the motions of cutting.

The youngster isn't actually allowed to cut hair for a while
but goes through the body movements. This helps to achieve
better mind and body co-ordination, so that, when she does
really start to cut hair, she doesn't feel all fingers and
thumbs.

There are many things to learn about cutting hair, for
example, a bad haircut shows visible scissor marks. These
are created when sections are left too thick (i.e. too much hair
is gathered together as a section), or the hair isn't wet down.
Sometimes I am afraid, it may be lack of interest on the
hairdresser's part. When I choose staff I try to choose
conscientious people who are happy in their work. I have
little time for miserable people. If they don't like hairdressing
then they should do something else. If we must spend about a
third of our lives working, then why not enjoy it?

Face shapes

One of the main arts of the hairdresser is to alter the
apparent shape of the face. We disguise the face shape by
varying the height, width and volume of different hairstyles.

OVAL

The oval is the easiest shape to add hairstyle to. The oval is
like an egg shape. Most styles suit the oval, unless there are
other problems to disguise such as a large nose or sticking out
ears, etc.

ROUND

I prefer to keep volume at the temples and top of the head,
to make the lower half of the face look thinner, and give the
style a more oval appearance. Hair swept onto the face can
help cover up the round look.

THIN

This needs more width to counteract the length. Again the idea is to try and make it look more like an oval. Long straight styles with no width make the face look even longer. Our eyes tend to follow lines of movement, so certain lines of movement can be exaggerated or toned down.

SQUARE

Soft movement is best to counteract the line of the square appearance. Think of the hairstyle as a picture and it's obvious that the square face can be made to look softer by adding the round movements of curls and waves. Have a rounded or feathered fringe, avoiding straight lines that emphasise the squareness.

BIG HEAD

The head looks larger when hair is short, revealing more head size. Make harsh features softer, using the methods appropriate for different head shapes.

LITTLE HEAD

The opposite applies here. If hair is left too long, the features look smaller, and the face becomes hidden within the hairstyle.

FOREHEADS

A high forehead is only emphasised by a high fringe. To alter this, the forehead should be covered in a soft manner.

A low forehead sometimes looks good covered up, because height and width can be added to the style to change the appearance.

NECKLINE

Long necks can be disguised with an appropriate hairstyle. Do not emphasise a long thin neck by cutting the hair too short. Do not make a fat neck look even fatter with a short shaped-in neckline. But make a short neck look longer with a well shaped hairstyle that draws attention to length at the nape.

SPECTACLES

If glasses are worn, they should be chosen to complement the features and hairstyle. Really large frames look out of place with a short shaped style. The spectacles should always harmonise with the style.

The above methods can be used to change the appearance or shape of certain features. However, there are sometimes less obvious points to take into consideration. Often square or even long features on a man look good. The square jawline looks masculine so it may be unnecessary to soften this face shape. Occasionally, prominent features help to give individual personality. A man may be noted for his overgrown eyebrows! Some fashionable styles don't always allow the hairdresser to try for a more oval finish, therefore you sometimes break the rules of hairdressing to achieve a different result.

Clothes are also important. They must suit the hairstyle and the shape of the body. Tall people with long thin features should avoid clothes with vertical lines (unless they want to look even taller) as they emphasise height. Broad people should avoid horizontal lines as they will add width.

Styles to suit you

Hairstylists begin their training by learning what styles suit which face shapes. As the stylist becomes more skilled, he/she learns that there are times to break the rules a little. You can see this from popular faces in magazines and on T.V. Many of them look nice, yet their hairstyles do not comply with the 'right' way that the hair should be styled for their face shape.

Hairstylists have different opinions as to what suits. It's important that you feel good about the way your hair is – confidence is the key. (Even when a new hairstyle looks wonderful on you, you can guarantee that someone won't like it! People have different tastes and of course they may prefer to see you with the same old style as before.)

Even the most awkward face shapes can take a great number of styles. The perfect shape for hairstyling is oval-faced. Usually most hairstyles suit this shape, but there are still many other considerations:

Height, figure, dress sense or individual style.

Complexion, features, ears, nose, mouth, etc.

Hair type, colour, movement, straight, curly, etc.

A good hairstylist can create a style and vary it to suit almost any type of face shape and features. The ever-changing fashion scene has some people following every fad regardless of whether the hairstyle or even clothes' style suits them or not.

Change isn't always such a bad thing. I change my own hairstyle regularly. A new hairstyle, one that suits you, can be very refreshing. Top hairstyling coupled with good use of make-up can bring about some amazing changes. With colour change as well, it's quite possible to look so different that your best friend won't recognise you! You may walk into a salon with a hairstyle you've had for years and walk out a different person. A good hairstyle can help give you confidence and uplift your spirits. It can do wonders for your personality. It's good to try new styles out sometimes.

I find that people are usually of two moulds: the doers and the watchers. The doers make mistakes of course, but they are exciting people. Life is a constant challenge for them. The watchers on the other hand are usually full of criticism, or perhaps praise, but they are reluctant to try anything new themselves. Sometimes they want to, but they lack self-confidence. Exciting styles usually have lots of movement – swept back off the face to emphasise features. Movement in a hairstyle helps to make a person look more dynamic. Sportsmen such as figure skaters often have their hair swept back in a flowing movement that blends in with the fast skating they do on the ice. Hairstyles may suit particular jobs, or are sometimes tailor-made to suit convention. Pop stars are expected to have flamboyant hairstyles but accountants and solicitors or M.P.s have a more traditional image to project.

Colour plays a large part in styling hair. Some colours blend well together, complementing each other. For ladies, hair colour must harmonise with make-up.

A very pale complexion looks terrible surrounded by a frame of black hair. The dark hair makes the pale skin stand out. This may be counteracted with make-up. Before colouring hair, take your stylist's advice, but make sure your hairdresser knows a lot about hair colour first. There is a wide selection of beautiful colours on the market. Of course if you have a lot of grey in your hair and you suddenly have a drastic colour change, you are asking for criticism. You would be better advised to tone the grey down a little, thus maintaining a natural appearance.

I often encourage our more "mature" clients to have more fashionable hairstyles. They say they would like to try a new style but feel they are much too old. I stress that I can make a variation of a modern style to suit the older lady. There is no reason why our more senior clients should walk out of the salon all wearing the same hairstyle. Sometimes they are even given a hairstyle that makes them look older!

Of course there are some styles that are strictly for the youngster mainly because of their shock impact. Often the weird styles created by pop stars are no more than cheap gimmicks to help them become noticed! Teenagers like to be different; it's exciting playing the rebel. Remember the old saying that you were young once yourself! Most of us have gone through that phase. Occasionally some great hairstyles come out of this and often the most shocking becomes fashionable later.

When choosing a new hairstyle, be a little daring. Look good – feel good. If you want to look younger, then choose a style that takes a couple of years off you, rather than one that puts years on. Confidence is the key. Most of us know someone who doesn't seem to age as quickly as the rest, but it's not because of some magic formula. The secret is partly in the mind. Once you start feeling old, then you are old.

The home hair tool kit

Here is what you need to look after your hair properly at home. In a sense, hair is like an item of clothing, but even more personal than that, so it's wise to invest in the right equipment to keep it looking good.

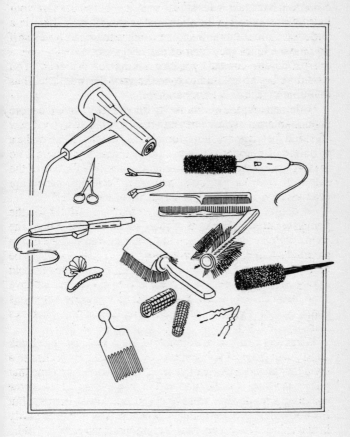

Fig. 16.   Necessary equipment.
Hairdryer, hairdressing scissors, hair clips, hot brush, pin tail comb, hairdressing tongs, normal hairdressing comb, hair grips, half backed brush, round brushes, afro comb, rollers and pins.

Hairdryer, one that is light and easy to handle, but reasonably powerful.

Pair of good sharp scissors for basic trimming in between visits to your local hairstylist.

Round brushes: large and small with soft bristles.

Combs: normal combing-out comb and possibly an afro for permed hair, and a tail or pin tail comb.

Half backed brush. I prefer a denman.

Hair grips to hold long hair up out of the way.

Hair tongs, hot brushes and *rollers.*

Hair gels, mousses and *fixing sprays.*

Hair lacquer, shampoo and *conditioners.*

Although quality articles may be quite expensive, if you become reasonably competent at blow-drying your own and your family's hair, you will save money.

Washing hair

Even among hairdressers, hair specialists and trichologists, there are conflicting opinions about washing hair. In my opinion, it should be washed regularly, and conditioned regularly, and it should be done properly.

I like a good thorough scalp massage when I have my own hair shampooed, I find it invigorating and refreshing, but hair type must be taken into consideration. If hair is fine and falling out, then care must be taken and hair should be shampooed gently. If hair is greasy, then a thorough scalp massage will only encourage the sebaceous glands to provide more natural oils, and thus make it worse.

For normal hair washing, two thorough shampoos are sufficient. You may use a shower or a basin with a bowl of water placed conveniently ready to rinse off the shampoo or conditioner. Comb all of your hair down from the nape, using a wide tooth comb to free any tangles. Make sure that all the hair is wet and then apply a lather all over the hair, not just in one spot. Use the balls of your fingers and massage all over the scalp using circular movements. Make sure the shampoo is rinsed off thoroughly and then start again. On rinsing the second time, you can check that the hair is clean by holding a piece of it tightly between your thumb and finger and pushing the hair up and down. This causes friction and the hair will squeak if it is wet and clean. Many hairdressers use this method to make sure all the shampoo is rinsed out.

Conditioners are for hair, not for scalp. Apply conditioner all over the hair, running it from roots to ends. Conditioners will do the scalp no good at all and may even block up the pores of the skin, causing spots. Some hairdressers believe that conditioners should only be left on for a couple of minutes. This may be all there is time for in the salon, but usually hair will be made softer and more manageable if the conditioner is left on longer. Check the instructions on the bottle – a basic conditioner can usually be left on the hair longer to do its job more thoroughly. But be careful with treatments that contain acids or peroxide; always follow the instructions exactly. If the instructions on a bottle of conditioner say it should be left on for five minutes, then it is wise to do this. When rinsing the conditioner off, make sure you rinse properly.

Most children seem to hate having their hair washed. Try to make it fun for them. Gently massaging their scalps can be very soothing. The same applies for husband and wife; you can take an interest in each other's welfare by shampooing each other's hair before blow-drying it into style.

A basic layer cut

I don't recommend that you cut your own hair. Even the best of hairstylists avoid this.

Some of the more adventurous of you might want to try a basic layer cut on your spouse, partner or your children. This cut is a variation which I have made easy to learn. If you follow each step carefully you should end up with a presentable style that will last at least until the next visit to a salon.

The layer cut is by far the most versatile hairstyle. It is equally suitable for men and women. It is the basis of a great number of hairstyle variations, so, if you are accomplished with this style, you will be able to cater for the whole family.

You need a sharp pair of scissors, of the same size that

your hairdresser uses. Proper hairdressing scissors can be
very expensive but they last a long time. They must be very
sharp to give an accurate cutting line, and of course care must
be taken not to cut yourself or the person involved.

Hair should be shampooed and left wet. Place a towel
around the person's neck and use a mirror placed in front of
you both so that you can judge length together.

Comb all tangles out of the hair and comb the hair (if
straight) flat to the skin. If the hair is curly, comb it as flat as
possible. Partings and breaks should only be added after the
cut but before the hair is blow-waved into place.

We will cut the base line (or perimeter) first. The base line
is the very edge of the hairstyle; the fringe, the base of the
sides and the hair at the lower part of the nape.

We then do the layers and this determines the actual
thickness and direction of the style. Layers can later be blow-
waved forward or back, or permed, etc., to create body and
the appearance of 'movement'.

The layers are checked by simply going over the cutting
process again and then cross-checked by standing at the side
of the hairstyle and simply picking a section up and looking to
see that there are no uneven ends.

The base line or edge of the hairstyle is checked again,
combing the hair down as straight and flat as possible once
more making sure that the cutting line is accurate.

If the hair is much longer than the desired length, cut some
of the excess length off first. Be careful that you leave enough
hair for the proper styling.

It is wise to follow the cutting pattern a couple of times
without actually cutting any hair off. If you go through all the
motions a few times, you'll feel more confident and more at
ease picking sections of hair up. When cutting children's
hair, extra care must be taken because they have a habit of
twitching about at the most unexpected times.

FRINGE

Stand at the front of the hairstyle and start by cutting one
half of the fringe. Hair shouldn't be pulled away from the skin
or this will cause graduation and it will be harder to get a good

cutting line; the eyes or eyebrows can be used as a guide to keep the fringe straight. Maintain hair tension but remember that when the hair is dry it will jump up slightly. Bend your knees to get your body down to see the style properly and keep good posture. Be extremely careful of the eyes, use part of your hand as a barrier between the eyes and your scissors. Never cut hair with one hand just dangling unused: use it to help steady the head or hold the hair and comb, or guide your scissors with it. Be very alert, don't take your eyes off what you're doing for a second. Remember how lethal a pair of scissors can be, look directly at the hair you're cutting.

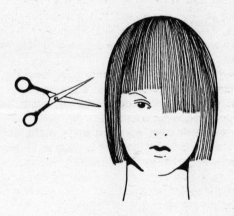

Fig. 17.   Cutting the first half of the fringe.

SIDE

When that half of the fringe is finished, stand at the side of the hairstyle. For the side we will cut the hair in a line going to the bottom of the ear lobe.

Fig. 18 shows the angle created so far. As the fringe slopes down, it curves slightly so that the cutting line doesn't look too severe. The hair is still kept close to the skin.

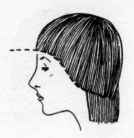

Fig. 18. Cut the hair in a line going to the bottom of the ear lobe.

OTHER SIDE OF FRINGE AND SIDE

Move around to the other side of the style and repeat the procedure, cutting the other half of the fringe and then down to the bottom of the ear lobe.

Check that both sides are even by stepping behind the hairstyle and making sure the head is straight. Drop yourself

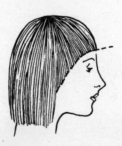

Fig. 19(a) The other side the same.

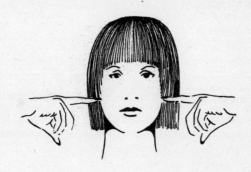

Fig. 19(b). Checking that both sides are even.

down to the level of the head and place a finger of each hand at earlobe level, as shown in fig. 19(b). Look in the mirror and make sure both sides are even. It's easy to imagine a line running from one finger to the other to give you a guide. Don't

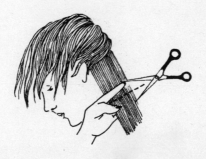

Fig. 20(a). Have the head bent down.

rely on the actual level of the ear lobes too much as many people have one ear lobe higher than the other. Rely more on your fingers being in line and horizontal.

REAR OF THE STYLE

Make sure the subject is sitting well back in the chair. This helps to keep the rest of the body straight and that is essential when trying for symmetry in the hairstyle. When cutting the rear of the style, it's important to make sure the head is bent down, revealing the nape as shown in fig. 20(a). Comb the hair flat against the skin and flatten with your finger, slide the scissors in gently and cut. The hair must be cut to blend with the sides and should still be reasonably wet.

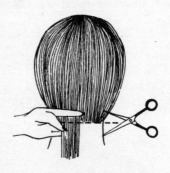

Fig. 20(b). Comb flat against the skin and flatten with your finger.

NOW WE HAVE THE PERIMETER

This will act as a guide line for the hairstyle, as can be seen in fig. 21. The hair within the perimeter will be cut in layers; when you start the layer cut, be careful not to thin the layers too much.

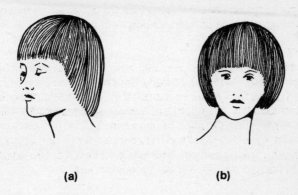

Fig. 21. The perimeter: **(a)** from the side; **(b)** full face.

CUTTING THE LAYERS

The head is divided into six parts, as shown in fig. 22, and hair is extended at a natural angle using very fine sections.

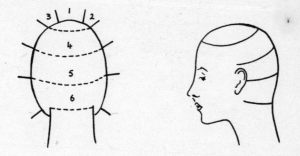

Fig. 22. The hair is divided into six parts.

PART ONE

For part number one, hair is raised and cut in sections from the front to the crown. Fig. 23(a) shows the sections used and their direction. Fig. 23(b) shows the angle that the haircut will follow, and Fig. 23(c) shows the cutting line.

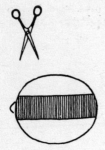

Fig. 23(a)
The sections used.

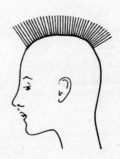

Fig. 23(b)
The angle.

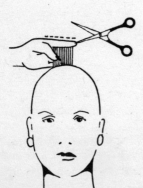

Fig. 23(c)
The cutting line.

PARTS TWO AND THREE

Parts numbers two and three are similar to each other. The cut goes from the front of the brow to the crown. Each section has a part of the previous section mingled in with it to give a guide line. This is shown in figs. 24 and 25.

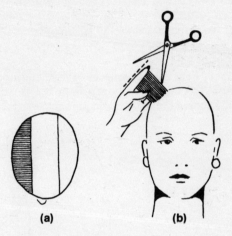

(a)   (b)

Fig. 24. Part number two:
(a) from above;   **(b)** showing the cutting line.

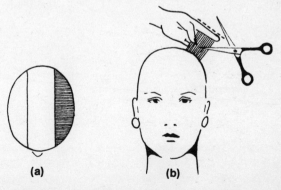

(a)   (b)

Fig. 25. Part number three:
(a) from above;   **(b)** showing the cutting line.

Whilst cutting hair at the sides, be aware of the type of hair your subject has got. If he is a man with a receding hairline at the temples, hair may be left slightly thicker. If hair is fine, covering the ears, be careful not to cut too much off revealing the ears through the hair. If he has a bald patch anywhere on the head, try to keep it covered. Leave hair at the crown slightly longer as the hair there has a tendency to stick up. Think about these things before the cut begins.

PART FOUR

This part goes right round the head and the cutting angle follows the contour of the head, as shown in fig. 26. Still use fine sections, keeping the tension. Be particularly careful at the ears.

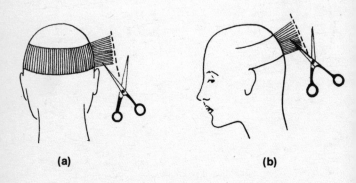

(a)   **(b)**

Fig. 26.   Part number four:
(a) from the rear;   **(b)** from the side.

PARTS FIVE AND SIX

Parts five (fig. 27(a) and (b)) and six (fig. 27(c) and (d)) are similar but the cutting angle can be changed to shape hair in at the nape. Some of these angles are awkward and may need some practice.

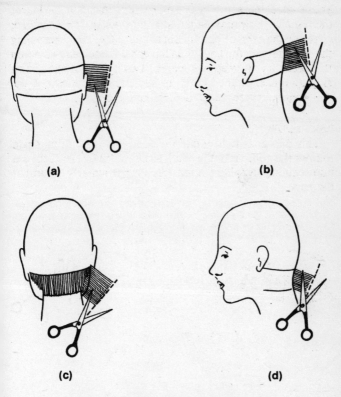

Fig. 27. **(a)** and **(b)** Part number five.
(c) and **(d)** Part number six.

When the layers are all cut, repeat the procedure to check over the cut you have completed. Hair should still be wet and fine sections should still be used. By reversing the cutting line you can cross-check the layers to make sure the cut is accurate. To do this, stand at the side of the hairstyle and pick hair up in the opposite direction to that used in cutting parts one, two and three. Just pick the sections up at random to check for any uneven pieces of hair.

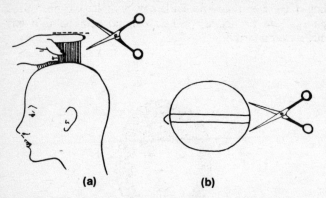

Fig. 28. Cross-checking: **(a)** the cutting line; **(b)** top view of cross section. By standing at the side, it is possible to take up sections of hair to check for any uneven pieces of hair.

Fig. 29 shows what the layers would look like if they stood up away from the head. It demonstrates the accuracy of the cut.

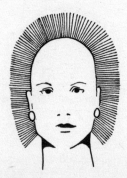

Fig. 29 The finished even layered cut. The diagram demonstrates an even cutting line if you imagine the hair standing away from the head.

Fig. 30 shows the cutting line you have used at the base line of the hairstyle. The cut is now complete. If need be, a parting can be added, or hair can be combed into any direction preferred.

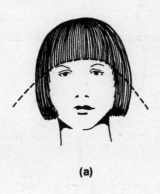

(a)

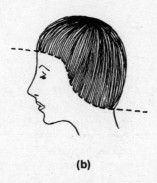

(b)

Fig. 30.   **(a)** This shows the rounded angle of the fringe.
(b) This shows the full cutting line of the perimeter.

Now the style can be blow-dried into shape with a round brush. This style is left quite natural so don't turn the base line under too tightly. At this stage hairspray can be used if necessary to keep the style looking good.

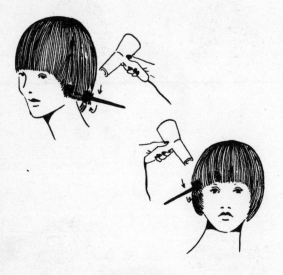

Fig. 31. Blow-drying the completed cut.

Cutting lines, fringe and sides

Here are a few examples of the many types of fringe and side shapes that can be cut into different styles.

Fringes can be tailored to individual needs, as shown in fig. 32.

The sides are an important part of the hairstyle, emphasising severe or soft features. Points, side boards and corkscrew curls, as well as those shown in fig. 33, are just a few examples.

There are many variations for fringe and side cutting lines. A good hairstylist will know a vast selection and can advise you more on suitable ones for your own features.

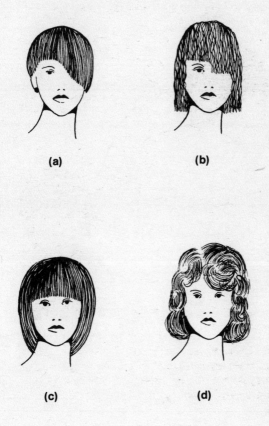

Fig. 32.   Fringes – showing variations of cutting angles.
(a) Asymmetric style – similar to a hat.
(b) Loosely permed.
(c) Short bob.
(d) Soft layered cut.

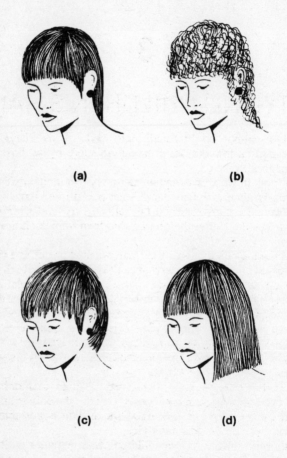

Fig. 33. Different sides.
(a) Very lightly feathered.
(b) Curly style.
(c) Feathered fringe and side.
(d) Square bob.

3

STYLING CHILDREN'S HAIR

Hair cannot be "trained" into style. It is changing, growing, falling out, and being affected by a host of influences every day.

If you have a reasonably short style and have it cut regularly, then within a year or so every hair will have been renewed. Perhaps it would be better to try and train our children to look after their hair rather than train the hair into style.

Many kids hate having their hair washed or cut and they can usually tell if the hairstylist can't be bothered with them. Having the wrong attitude when cutting children's hair merely encourages a similar response. Usually even the hysterical child can be talked round and calmed by a patient, caring hairdresser. To a child, scissors can look menacing and the other tools such as electric clippers must look as if they're going to chop a kid's head off. It's up to the hairstylist to make children feel at ease.

Children often turn up with all sorts of tangles in their hair, and even chewing gum and sweets. Usually the only solution is to cut the gum out, leaving as much hair as possible to maintain some kind of hairstyle.

It's very difficult to keep children's hair in good condition because of the hectic lifestyle they lead, but kids are becoming fashion-conscious at a very early age now, so it pays to try. I find very young kids looking through style books nowadays. More little children have perms and highlights now as well. If you encourage them to take an interest in their own hair, it will take some of the heat off you, and you'll find them sitting in front of the mirror combing their hair into place at a very early age. The next few pages deal with some of the popular children's hairstyles and methods of keeping them looking neat. Eventually, as they grow older, they will be familiar with blow-waving methods themselves.

The following styles are suitable for adults as well as children. I have selected a few that are really ideal for kids mainly because they are easy to style. They are no problem to keep looking good, smart, and clean and they never seem to leave the fashion scene.

Most Mums with busy schedules need styles for their children that are very easy to manage. Styles that look smart help to stimulate children's interest in looking after their own appearances. In the salon I have seen proof of this many times. We give a child a more interesting hairstyle and when Mum visits us again she is amazed at how her child has suddenly started to groom the style into shape before going to school or the local disco. This applies to boys as well as girls.

More kids are now using gel and mousses on their hair and there is a definite increase in the number of children who want fashionable hairstyles.

The following hairstyles should be ideal:

Straight bobs

For short bobs that are simply turned under, keep the dryer pointing downwards, but not directly into the scalp. Turn the hair under with a small round brush or a half backed styling brush. Dry the roots, then middle lengths, then ends, turning the hair tightly under. For thick hair, section the hair up. If finishing with tongs (see p.68) or heated brush, remember not to leave hair in the heat for too long. A good way of ensuring this is to count 'one, two, three', whilst holding the hair in the tongs and then move on to tong the next piece of hair – this makes sure that you don't damage the hair at all.

Always remember, dry out excess water from hair first as this saves a lot of time. If your child has a parting, you may use a comb to style the parted hair, following the movement of the comb with the dryer.

The bob is easy to style this way as all the hair is blow-dried down and turned under at the bottom. Be careful not to tangle the hair in the brush. Be extra careful not to turn the hairdryer round the wrong way, thus sucking hair into the back of the dryer. This is a common fault of beginners. It is not only dangerous, but also disastrous to the style, as usually the only way to free the tangle is to cut the hair off.

The straight bob is ideal for most straight styles but remember with boys not to turn the hair under too much, otherwise the hairstyle may look rather effeminate.

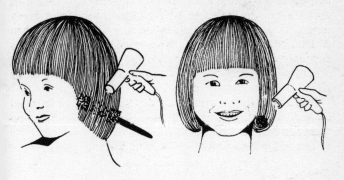

Fig. 34. A straight bob.

Flicked bob

For styles that are flicked away from the face, the blow-drying method is practically the opposite to the last style although the cut may be very similar.

Turn the hair around the brush but this time outwards from the head. Blow the hair from underneath, as shown in fig. 35. This works better with wavy hair but if your child's hair is straight then apply blow-dry lotion or mousse to help maintain the style. For a really smart look, use the tongs to curl the hair outwards. A soft perm also helps if the hair has little movement of its own. Don't hold the hairdryer too close to the hair or keep it pointed at one spot for too long or this will dry the hair out, causing split ends and making it brittle. Lots of variation can be made by just flicking one half out or even just the fringe. Experiment with it.

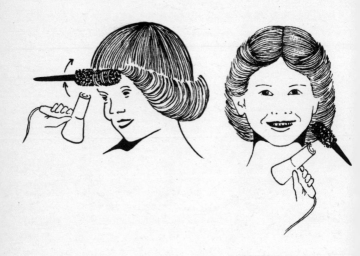

Fig. 35. Flicked bob.

Layered cut blown back

This style is very versatile, basically blowing hair from the front to the back, top and sides. It has many variations depending on the length, sometimes it is brought down onto the brow and then blown back, sometimes the sides are brought down and the top is swept back. For this variation, pull the hair tight around the brush and then take it back in stages from the brow. It usually requires medium-length layers all over. For girls, it's usually given more volume or body, and movement. For boys, not too much volume. If the hair is cut shorter on top a spiky variation is created. Sometimes a loose perm may be required to create movement in the hair.

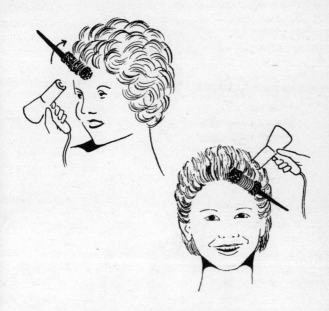

Fig. 36.   Layered cut blown back.

Short hair with side parting

If the hair is very short a little force may be required to control it. The brush or comb simply directs the hair flat, followed by the dryer blow-waving the hair into style. Dry the parting first. Otherwise you could lose it when drying the rest of the style.

This style is always popular for children as well as for grown-ups because it's so easy to keep looking neat.

Very strong hair tends to spike up if cut short, so make sure you know exactly what you want when you cut it. Remember that if hair is very short it will be impossible to perm. No volume is required with this sort of hairstyle.

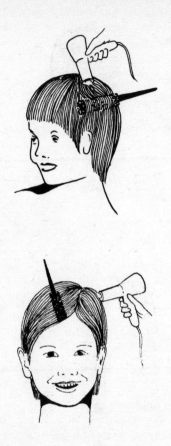

Fig. 37. Short hair with side parting.

Drying really long hair

For long hair you will need hair grips. Dry out excess
moisture and then section the hair up out of the way, as in fig.
38(a). We will start at the back of the head. Dry the roots first
and then follow the brush through the hair with the dryer.

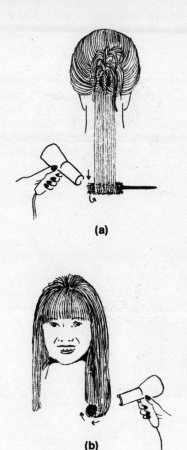

Fig. 38. Drying really long hair.

Again, don't point hot air at the scalp; always point it at the hair, but keep it moving up and down the hair shaft.

Drying long hair is time-consuming, but you can speed it up by using the same methods as are used by professionals.

At the ends, the hair is turned under. Do one section at a time. Dry each section thoroughly. Then the hair can be tonged.

Tonging method

Most hairdressing tools work on similar principles. The set is similar to a perm and the blowstyle is similar to the set because the round brush is nothing more than a roller with a handle on the end of it. Tongs are a bit like perm rods. Hair is trapped around the rod and the heat forms a wave in the hair. If the tongs are left on for too long the heat will damage the hair. A simple rule to apply is to place the hair around the tongs and count 'one, two, three', then move on to tong the next piece of hair. This ensures that the tongs don't damage the hair.

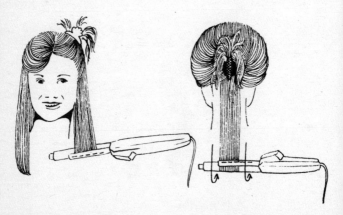

Fig. 39. Tonging method.
(Section clips have been used to keep some of the hair out of the way.)

For this blowstyle, the tonging method we will use requires the hair to be sectioned again now that it is dry and each section is tonged under. Make sure that the ends of the hair aren't buckled (this also applies to sets and perms etc.). The hair from the ends is rolled smoothly around the tongs and trapped there until the heat does its job and a stronger curl is created. This style is one length, not layered at all. Only the middle lengths and the ends of the hair need be tonged. Go all the way round the head, making a smooth tight finish. Be careful not to lie the tongs on the scalp; if necessary, place your comb between the tongs and the scalp as a guard. You should create a nice tucked-under effect.

If hair is damp when you use the tongs, the style will not look as good. This is a mistake made by some beginners. Drying long hair is a very long job for the inexperienced; with practice it becomes easier and faster.

4

STYLING MEN'S HAIR

Over the last few years short- and medium-length hair has been the trend for most men. Short hair for men will continue to be fashionable because it is easier to keep smart and clean, and convenient for busy work schedules or sports that work up a sweat. Fashion changes, but in general the trend seems to be for ladies to keep their hair longer than gentlemen.

The use of the hairdryer by men first thing on a morning before going off to work, or before a night out, has risen tremendously. The days when all men had practically identical haircuts are over. It's vital to look good in most jobs these days, and hairstyle is therefore of the utmost importance.

The following pages show a few blowstyling methods that ladies can use to groom their partners' hair. Try them out. I'm sure that you'll find them interesting, as well as being good fun and a possible money-saver.

Short swept back style with parting

This gentleman's style is cut short around the ears and shaped in. The fringe and layers are left long so that there is enough length to sweep back. The style is parted.

This kind of style needs no volume. It is turned under around the brush gently without adding body or lift, as shown in fig. 40. When it is dry, it is swept back from the fringe. The back is blown flat at the nape. This hairstyle is always fashionable; it has been around in one form or another for a long time.

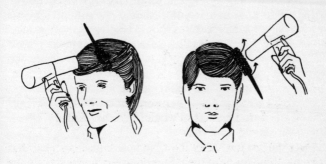

Fig. 40.   Short swept back style with parting.

Swept back style without parting

Another popular style. It is similar to the parted style but now we use the round brush to curl the hair back off the face. This gives the hairstyle more volume than the parted style. The hair may need a loose perm to soften it and help the blow-waving method.

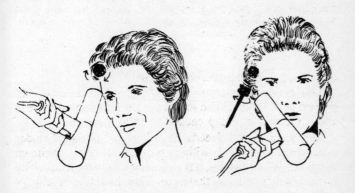

Fig. 41.   Swept back without parting.

Gentleman's feathered style

Gentlemen's hairstyling follows different rules from that of ladies' styling. Harsh features should be softened where necessary, but gentle features should be given a more macho image. If the style needs to be softened, do not make it look too feminine. Men's styles don't need much body or movement.

This style is more like a feathered cut, at least at the fringe. Again don't create much volume or tuck the hair underneath around the perimeter. This would lose the feathery effect. The style should look natural.

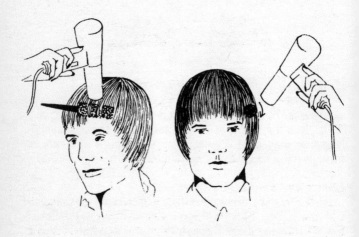

Fig. 42. Gentleman's Feathered style.

Some movement is necessary. Create it by blowing the hair not too tightly around a small round bristle brush. Again, lotions can be used to help keep the shape, although some hair won't need any. Do one section after another, using the brush all over. Balance the volume evenly around the head, otherwise hair will stick up higher in some places and seem to be flat in others.

Centre parted style, blow-waved back at sides

This style is cut in layers, short and close at the sides but left fairly long at the back, just hanging over the collar. This is a popular gentleman's style.

Don't add a lot of volume. With most hair types, the hair can be turned under with a round brush first, before it is swept back.

This hairstyle looks great with highlights to emphasise movement, or a soft perm to create a different image.

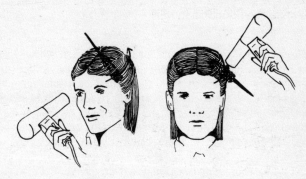

Fig. 43. Centre parted style.

Beards and moustaches

History has featured a multitude of different types of beard and moustache. Most of these styles have all but died out. Fig. 44 shows some of the styles that are sometimes seen in films which try to capture the era when they were considered trendy. Some of these styles can still be seen from time to time, and no doubt as the wheel of fashion turns they will become popular once more.

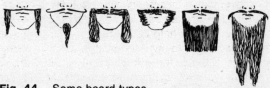

Fig. 44. Some beard types.

Many of them had names such as forked or goatee beards or walrus or handlebar moustaches. I'm sure you can pick them out.

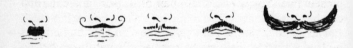

Fig. 45. Some moustache types.

Remember if your husband, or the gentleman whose hair you are styling, has a beard, it should be styled to complement his hair. A man should not have his hair cut short and leave a long thick beard which looks out of place with the new overall shape. Any good stylist would recommend that the beard is toned down to suit the hairstyle. This should apply to the sideburns and moustache as well.

Not only should the beard match the hairstyle but also the hairstyle should match the height, figure and other characteristics. For example, if a man is small and he has a mass of hair, it will make him look even smaller.

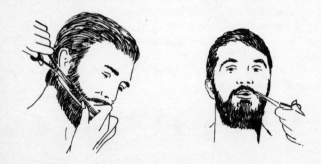

Fig. 46. Trimming a beard.

Beard trimming

Many ladies enjoy trimming their partner's beard or moustache. This method is quite easy. Although it won't line and style the beard, it will keep it thinned out and looking presentable. You need a sharp pair of scissors and a normal comb.

The comb is placed flat against the skin and the hair that protrudes through its teeth is trimmed. Be careful to decide exactly how short you want the beard to be. The thickness of the teeth of the comb will determine the length of the beard and act as a barrier between the skin and the scissors.

5

STYLING WOMEN'S HAIR

More and more men now blow-dry and style their partner's
hair. It is reasonably easy to learn.

The styles that follow are related to the men's styles in the
previous chapter. They differ mainly in terms of the amount
of movement, and the volume involved.

Swept back style

Remember to dry out excess water first with the towel, and
then use the hairdryer with finger or brush. This saves a lot of
time, especially on long hair.

This style is similar to the man's swept back style on page
71. The hair may either be turned under at the back, or
curled up and around the brush and blow-waved from each
side of the head towards the middle, similar to the d/a
neckline style. Hair should be blow-waved tightly around the
brush in sections and tonged when it is thoroughly dried.
Don't tong damp hair. It makes a mess of the style. The brush
should create little rolls all over the head. Usually ladies'
styles need a little more time spent on the blow-drying and
combing out at the end.

Feathered style

This ladies' style is a contrast to the men's feathered style,
as we follow different rules for ladies' blow-drying.

The style is cut into a wispy feathered finish and the hair is
swept and blow-dried around the head onto the face from
right to left. The right side is brought forward and the left side is

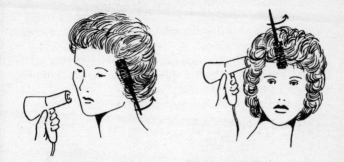

Fig. 47. Swept back style
    (a) Blow-drying the left-hand side of the hairstyle.
    (b) Blow-drying the front of the hairstyle.

brought back, so that the hair is swept round the crown of the head like a whirlpool. The base line must not be turned under too tightly or it will lose its feathered finish. The style is given a lot of body with the round brush, using sections all over following the spiral movement. Finish by using tongs, but not around the perimeter. Quite a lot of practice is needed to make this work really well.

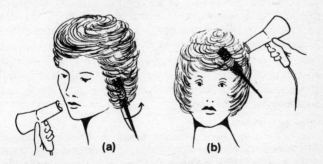

Fig. 48. Variations of a lady's feathered style.
(a) Hair is swept around the crown with the round brush like a whirlpool.
    The right side is swept forward and the left side is swept back.
(b) The hair is swept onto the face.

The swept back and feathered styles can also be finger-dried using the fingers as a movable comb or brush to give a natural finish with lots of movement. Using your fingers teaches you how to move the dryer correctly, because if the heat is being directed at one place for too long the hot air will burn your fingers slightly before it has a chance to damage the hair. Eventually you will move the dryer properly and not burn your fingers or damage the hair or scalp.

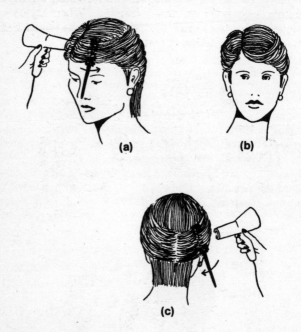

Fig. 49. Flicked back style.
The hair is swept back and then towards the middle at the rear. The hair is not built out away from the head. Lift or volume has not been added to the roots.

Flicked back style
   This style can be flicked back either at one side or at both sides, depending on preference. There are many variations of

it. If the hair has waves, then it can be flicked out around the brush. Hair without waves may be cut with graduation or layers, and it is turned under first before being combed back into shape (fig. 49(a)). This style is flicked back at the sides, cut short with points in front of the ears, and shaped in at the nape.

Hair at the sides is wound around the brush and blown up and back around the brush, creating movement (fig. 49(c)). The hair at the back is blown down without adding lift. Styles like this look good on small features. When styled on someone with a large head, the hair needs to be longer, to be in harmony with the larger features.

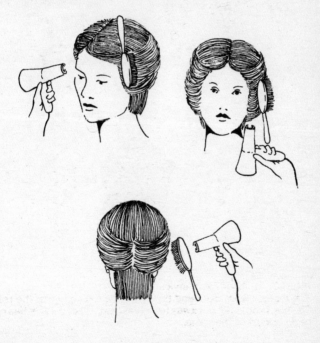

Fig. 50. Graduated style.
The hair is flicked back and into the middle at the rear. This style has more volume than the previous one.

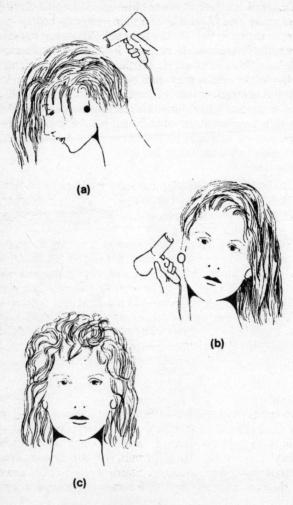

Fig. 51. Wild style
(a) Bend the head down.
(b) Blow-dry into the roots.
(c) The wild style complete.

Graduated style

This graduated style may be blow-dried smoothly from the roots to the middle lengths and then gently flicked up at its base, as shown in fig. 50. The haircut holds its style position very well. When it is cut properly it looks very impressive, with the graduation showing off the contrasting movement. Variations in colour may also be added to the style. For example, the underneath hair may be coloured dark which gives a good contrast when flicked up into position. Very short graduated styles need to be cut regularly to keep their shape.

Wild style

This style is very popular and features the scrunch drying method. Scrunch drying is done exactly as it sounds. Hair is scrunched between the fingers and dried, adding lots of body and volume with the hairdryer.

Volume can be added to the roots by combing all the hair up and blow-drying into it. Another method is to bend the head right down, as in fig. 51(a), and add volume this way. Put lots of body up through the roots to make the hair stand out and scrunch it together. When the head is straight again and the hair is dried properly, the volume you have added will make the hair stand out in a wild style, full of movement. The hair must be cut in reasonably long layers. Gel and mousse or fixing spray all help to keep the hair in place.

Spiked styles

Spiked styles are a typical example of unisex styling and look equally good on men or women. The spike will always be in fashion in one form or another. Such famous spiky hairstyles were the Rod Stewart, or the David Bowie hairstyle used during his Ziggy Stardust phase. Then there's the shorter variation popular for men or women, the flat top.

Spiky hair can be worn with or without a fringe – with long or short perimeter hair. These styles work well on reasonably strong hair. Fine hair has to be gelled so that it will stand up.

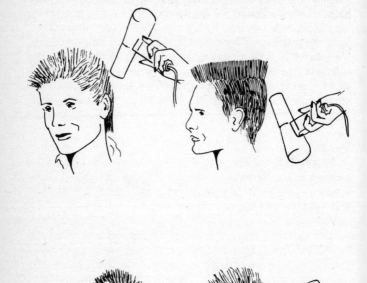

(c)   (d)

Fig. 52.   A selection of unisex spiky styles.
(a) Short, neat and slightly spiky.
(b) Flat top hairstyle.
(c) and **(d)** Spiky styles can be gelled and left messy or made to stand right up on top.

Strong hair stands up easily because when it is short, its natural direction is upwards.

Simply apply gel if necessary and brush and blow-dry the hair from the back to the front.

6

STYLING WEST INDIAN, ASIAN AND AFRICAN HAIR

One of the most eye-catching things about Indian, African and Oriental hair is the quality, the glossy shine and the thick rich texture. Some styles which look very ordinary on a white person look superb when cut into this dark glossy hair.

For ladies, if the hair is straight and to be kept in a one length style such as a pageboy, the cutting line must be accurate. A good cutting line stands out particularly well and the naturally shiny hair will show off the style admirably. If the hair is in good condition it will often have a pleasant silky feel to it.

For men it's very important to get the layers cut right. The hair must be wet. The emphasis on fine sections is crucial here because this type of hair shows up any mistakes much more clearly. The basic layer cut shown on page 45 is suitable for straight black hair, with the following adaptations:

The cut must be checked and double checked, because mistakes show up more clearly.

Finer sections must be used because the hair is usually thicker, and scissor marks will show up as faint lines within the hairstyle.

Generally the hair is more brittle and the cutting line stands out more.

The hair should be conditioned before cutting to make it soft and silky, and therefore easier to manage.

The hair may be permed or coloured but care should be taken. Hairdressing is full of surprises. Sometimes hair that looks very strong and thick will perm or colour very quickly. This is especially so with Chinese or Japanese types.

Straight Indian and Oriental hair types have a lot in common. Beginners often refer to this as 'hair like wire'. But the more experienced hairdresser gets a feel for this hair, and adapts to its different texture.

A few years ago I remember attending a hair-colouring competition. At this particular one I wasn't actually taking part, but it was interesting to watch. One style stood out from the rest, this was a dark model whose hair had been bleached and then coloured. The result was quite startling because of the colour contrast. The usually dark hair had a mixture of blonde shades and bright reds and was very eye-catching. Even though it wasn't placed highly in the competition, I will never forget it. It showed how versatile hair can be in the hands of an adventurous stylist with exciting ideas about cutting, perming, and colouring.

I would advise all coloured people to be particularly careful when visiting a salon for the first time. Your hair needs the attention of a specialist familiar with Indian, African, and Oriental hair.

Afro cut

Sometimes dark frizzy hair seems very thick. In reality each individual hair may be fine, although there may be a lot of hair on the head. If the hair is tight and curly, it may look a lot shorter than it is when it is stretched out.

The following diagrams show a cutting method used to style afro hair. You will need an afro comb, a normal comb, and a pair of sharp scissors.

The method used will depend on the tightness of the curl. If the hair isn't a true afro and hasn't got a lot of tight curls, then the normal layer cut can be used.

If the hairstyle is a true curly afro, this is an easy method to follow:

Comb the hair up and out with the afro comb all over the head as shown in fig. 53, missing none out. You will find the volume increases as the curls are loosened and pulled up. You will find a lot of hair hidden because the curls are so tight.

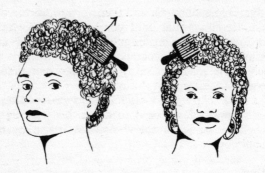

Fig. 53.   Comb the hair up and out with the afro comb.

Now with scissors and a normal comb begin to cut off the excess length as shown in fig. 54. The cut goes around the contour of the style and this is what you are aiming for, *a new contour.*

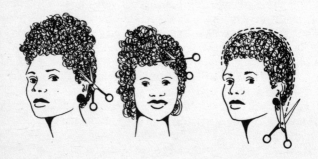

Fig. 54.   Hair has been combed out with an afro comb. Now the contour is cut.

Work on this until you are satisfied with the new contour. Then start all over again pulling the hair up and out with the afro comb once more. You will find a lot more hair still crinkled up in the curls.

Cut the excess off again and then go through the whole process once more still, until you are satisfied with the contour. You must work on this until it is perfect. You can see the cutting contour more accurately if you place a large white card behind the head (fig. 55(b)). The black hair shows up better against the card.

In the salon, clippers are often used to achieve the same result, and scissors are used to finish the style off. But scissors can be used to do the whole style when clippers are unavailable.

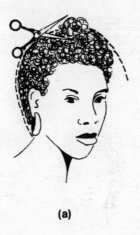

(a)

Fig. 55.
(a) Every piece of hair is cut to perfection.

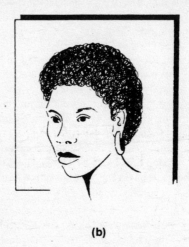

(b)

Fig. 55.
(b) The afro complete showing a perfect contour.

7

SETTING, PERMING AND SPECIAL EFFECTS

A basic set

When setting hair you must follow the natural movement of hair growth. The hair must be wet. It is pulled up at the angle shown in fig. 56(a), using the tail of a tail comb, and wound around the rollers in sections. Sections are taken from the front of the head and rolled towards the back. The hair must be stretched and wound tightly around the rollers, making sure that the ends aren't buckled, or the result will be frizzy. The sections should be thin so that the hair is set into place without gaps appearing, or straight hair showing through on the combing in.

Thinner rollers are used near the nape and hairline to follow the contour of the style. In the salon, the hair is dried under a large stationary dryer. At home, you could use a hood dryer, or just leave it to dry naturally. Setting lotion or mousse can be used and a net is usually placed over the rollers to maintain the style and stop the rollers from falling out. When the hair is dry, if it has been set tightly without gaps it will comb in very easily. A half backed brush is used to comb the style through and then the tail comb to finish the style off. There may be a break at the front to give a half fringe, or alternatively the style may go straight back.

Setting can achieve some attractive styles and the ability to put rollers in properly is essential. A similar pattern is used for some perms.

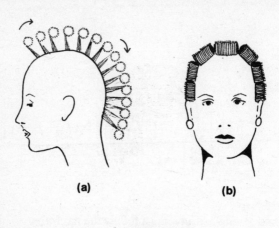

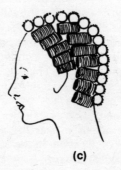

Fig. 56.
(a) The direction that the rollers are wound into place.
(b) The rollers set to sweep hair back off the face.
(c) A popular setting pattern.

Pin curling at home

Pin curling has a variety of uses. One of the commonest is for the fringe, or other parts of a set, to give a different and smaller curl. For the pin curl used in figs. 57 and 58, the hair

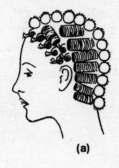

(a)

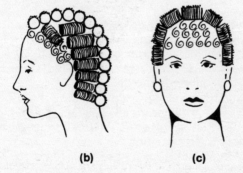

(b)   **(c)**

Fig. 57.   Pin curls in the perimeter of a set.
(a) The pin curl clips are still in the style.
(b) and **(c)** The pin curl clips have been removed to show the
angle of the curl that has been set into place, using two slightly
different setting patterns.

is cut in medium-length layers. It must be wet when pin curled and then it will dry into the curled shape. Plastic pins are the best type if you are using a home hood dryer, because the metal ones can become very hot.

Attempt a few individual pin curls first before trying to do a whole style with them. Fig. 58 shows the *pin curl movement.*

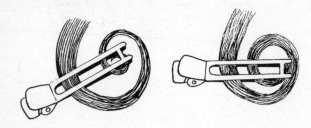

Fig. 58.   This shows the pin curl movement.

The ends of the hair are trapped under the clip and they are dried into position thus forming the curl. Experiment putting pin curls into the perimeter hair when you do a set, as suggested in fig. 57. This creates soft waves, and is an ideal way of giving movement to the hair.

Now try to do a whole style using pin curls. In the first style (fig. 59(a) and (b)) the curls all go the same way, but in the second (fig. 59(c) and (d)), the movement is changed halfway up the head to give an attractive wavy contrast.

It is even possible to perm hair using pin curls. In some salons they are used to complement blowstyling, but in others their use is virtually nil. This is a shame. Each head of hair is different, and hairdressers should employ every technique that is available.

Perming hair

To curl hair we stretch and wind it around a perm rod and then add a perm lotion, or, to use the correct term, reagent. Basically the perm changes the structure of the cortex.

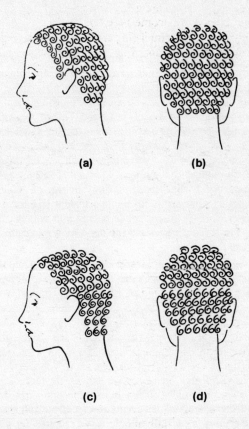

Fig. 59. In these diagrams the pin curl clips have been removed, revealing the pin curls set into place before they are combed into style.

(a) and **(b):** This pin-curling method creates a movement one way.

(c) and **(d):** Here we can create a contrasting movement by placing pin curls the opposite way halfway down the head.

There are linkages inside the hair that form its shape. The perm lotion breaks these down whilst the hair is stretched around the roller. The neutraliser is then applied, building up new linkages and thus creating the new hair shape. These linkages are called disulphide linkages and if they aren't built up properly the hair will be damaged.

To keep your perm looking smart it should be conditioned regularly. Leave the conditioner on for a few minutes and then comb through with a normal comb after rinsing, then comb through with an afro comb to free the curls.

Hair should never be conditioned before a perm. The conditioner covers the hair in a protective barrier, which stops the perm from soaking through into the cortex.

Blow-drying, perming and setting are all similar procedures. They each change the shape of the hair. They create a new contour around the head, giving height or volume or movement to a hairstyle. By using different size rods we can make very tight perms or loose perms and waves.

Here are the commonest reasons why some perms don't take properly:

Hair sections too thick.
Perm not left on the hair long enough.
Hair is already damaged before it is permed.
Perm is left on for too long.
Rods incorrect size for the desired effect.
Ends are buckled when hair is wound round rod.
Two people wind rods and one winds tighter sections than the other.
Hair has been badly cut.

All of these reasons, and others, can affect the result of a perm. Perming is a skill which is only learnt by practical experience. Once you find a hairdresser with this type of experience, stick with that hairdresser.

A basic perm
Most perms smell because of the ammonia content, although some modern ones don't smell as bad.

While the perm rods and the type of perm determine the

tightness and lasting effects of the perm, all sorts of things can be used to perm hair, even chopsticks or pipe cleaners! New ways of perming are constantly being created and hair can be permed on virtually anything that it can be wound round.

A perm can be used to soften strong hair giving wave or body, or hair may be just partly permed to create an asymmetric style.

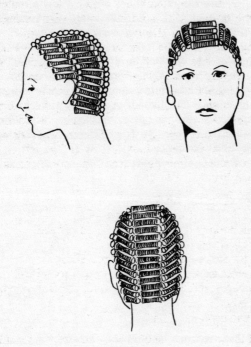

Fig. 60.   A completed perm showing the position and angle of perming rods.

The perming style in fig. 60 is the most common. It follows the same angle as a basic set and the natural growth angle of the hair. Hair is divided into very fine sections and pulled tight but not so tight as to cause discomfort for the person involved. The ends of the hair are smoothed. The paper is folded in half and the ends of the hair are trapped in the fold, then wound to the roots around the perm rod. Many hairdressers apply the perm lotion to the hair as they wind the perm but some apply the lotion when the whole perm is wound. Then a plastic bag is placed over the top of the head to cover the perm rods.

Depending on hair type, the perm lotion is left on for about 5 to 20 minutes, but it is important if using a home perm to read and follow the instructions completely. Instructions vary; some say 5 to 15 minutes, etc. When ready, the perm is rinsed carefully and then – leaving the rods in – the neutraliser is applied. Cotton wool can be placed around the hairline to stop the chemical dripping. Neutraliser is frothed up and applied all over the perm rods thoroughly. This may be left on for 5 to 10 minutes. The rods may be taken out then and the neutraliser can be applied again and left on for a couple of minutes. This procedure may be slightly different for some products and again it is important to follow the directions on the bottle. For different hairdressing products there are different methods. If you find that a perm is taking a long time to create its curl then you must leave the perm lotion on a little longer than the instructions suggest, but check it every couple of minutes so that it doesn't become over-processed.

The finished perm may be blow-dried, set, left to dry naturally, or perhaps scrunch dried with the fingers.

If you want to perm your hair at home and are worried that the perm might harm your hair, carry out a test first. Snip a little hair off – enough to be wound around the perm rod – perhaps during a normal haircut. If your whole hairstyle doesn't need to be cut at the time, just cut a little hair from the style. Don't just cut a chunk from anywhere. You could take it from the back or perhaps from underneath the main length of hair. You don't need much and if the hair is reasonably long you can easily snip it off without making it apparent that it has been cut. Don't cut the hair right down to the roots, try to leave a couple of inches to blend into the style. If the hair is too short to do this, it may be too short to perm anyway. Then, wind the hair like any normal perm and go through the correct procedure, applying perm lotion, rinsing after the required time and then neutralising.

If a perm is done incorrectly or over-processed it could make the hair very dry or snap it or even turn it into a frizzy mess! But there should be no need to worry if the instructions are followed carefully.

Perm rod sizes

Fig. 61 shows what curl size can be achieved from different rod sizes. The smaller rods will produce tight curly perms. As the rods get larger a looser perm will result. This latter sort of perm will simply add body and wave to a style. For some parts of the head, a mixture of rod sizes is used to achieve the desired result.

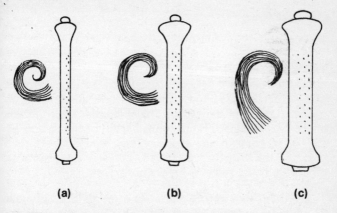

     (a)   **(b)**   **(c)**

Fig. 61.   Different rod sizes and the curls they produce.
(a) Tight. (Curly perm.)
(b) Medium. (Perm to add body to style.)
(c) Soft. (Loose perm to hang soft and natural or add movement.)

Fig. 62 shows the stages in winding a perm rod. When the perm has been wound and left to take, the hairdresser should check regularly to see that the curl is forming properly. This is done by unwinding a rod slightly. Without letting the hair escape, tension is relaxed a little and the curl that has formed will take shape. When the perm has taken, the hair should be rinsed thoroughly before the neutraliser is applied.

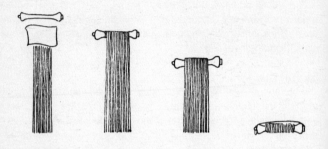

Fig.62. Winding the hair round the perming rods, showing the rod, paper and hair.

Perm types

STACK PERM

This style is cut in long layers and then the hair is permed using different-sized rods. The perimeter of the style is permed tightly, the middle parts more loosely, while the hair on the top of the head is not permed at all. Each rod rests on the one underneath and as the perm is wound looser each time, the stacked effect is created. The rest of the perming procedure is the same as for the basic perm.

The perm rods can be put around the head in different directions to produce different directions of curl movement. Obviously in a book of this length I can't cover every type of perm in detail, but figures 64 and 65 illustrate two more perm types you may come across.

WEAVE PERM

This type of perm is usually done on reasonably long hair. It gives a softer more natural finish, leaving sections of the hair straight and others curly.

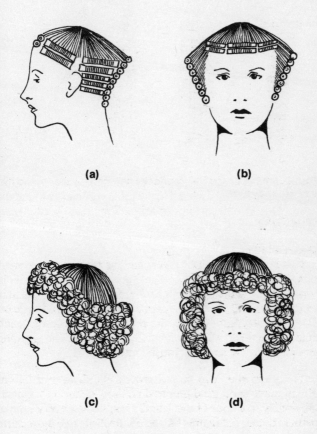

Fig. 63. Stack perm.
(a) Side view showing the perm rods.
(b) Front view showing the perm rods.
(c) Side view of completed perm.
(d) Front view of completed perm.

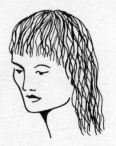
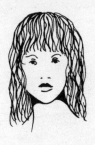

Fig. 64.   Weave perm.

SPIRAL PERM

The perm rods are wound to the roots vertically around the head. This also needs hair of reasonable length and gives a lovely corkscrew curl finish.

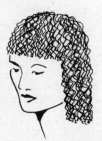
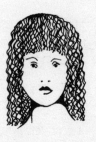

Fig. 65.   Spiral perm.

PERMING PARTS OF A STYLE

The whole head of hair needn't be all permed. An effective style is produced by perming just one side of the head or the back. The hairstyle should be designed for this. Fig. 66

shows a few examples of styles where only parts of the hairstyle are permed.

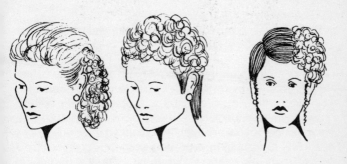

Fig. 66.   Perming parts of a hairstyle.

Basic colour knowledge

Whether you intend to apply a home product or visit your local hair salon it is essential to know a little about the different types of hair colouring. There are three basic types:

(i)   Temporary colours, mousses, setting lotions, rinses, etc.

(ii) Semi-permanent colours, colour baths, rinses, etc.

(iii) Permanent tints, of which there is a vast selection.

(i)   TEMPORARY COLOUR

Washes out very quickly. It merely coats the cuticle without affecting the pigment in the cortex of the hair. This sort of colouring is handy for party nights out, when you fancy being a little different but want your normal colour back for the next day.

(ii) SEMI-RINSES

These colours are meant to wash out after half-a-dozen to a dozen shampoos, depending on the condition of your hair.

They are usually the first step towards having a permanent tint, and a good way of trying colour out. The colour gets deeper into the hair cuticle.

(iii) PERMANENT TINTING

There is a wide variety of makes of tint and often the tint looks so professional that even an expert might have trouble spotting it!

Tint is mixed with hydrogen peroxide so that the colour can go right into the colour pigment in the cortex. Remember that re-growth will be a bit of a problem and it will be necessary to re-tint regularly to keep the roots balanced with the tinted hair. If you are applying colour yourself you will be amazed at how quickly your roots need doing, especially if the colour you have chosen is in strong contrast to the natural colour.

Basically, colour exists in hair because of pigment. Pigments within the cortex absorb and reflect light to certain degrees. We call these different colours 'the colour spectrum'. If hair absorbs only a few of the colours of the spectrum it will be lighter. The more colours of the spectrum it absorbs, the darker it will be. If hair reflects just one colour of the colour spectrum then it will appear to be that colour.

When we add artificial colour to hair we are adding pigments that absorb or reflect the colours of the colour spectrum. On the other hand when we bleach hair, or add highlights, we are actually taking colour out.

In both cases there is a need for hydrogen peroxide. If applying a dark colour to hair then a weak percentage of hydrogen peroxide is used. For example, when colouring brown hair very dark or black we would use 3% hydrogen peroxide (10 vol.).

If we needed to make the brown hair a couple of shades lighter – say light brown or dark blonde – we would add the necessary tint to a higher percentage hydrogen peroxide (9%/30 vol.). If we wanted to highlight brown hair we would need to add 9% or 12% (30 or 40 vol.) to bleach the hair. So the rule here is the lighter you want the hair to become – the stronger the peroxide percentage.

We can remove the natural colour from hair with bleach until it loses all of its colour. The hair colour will change from dark to the blonde used for highlights and, if left on longer, it will eventually go white. If we wanted to turn dark brown hair into a very light red shade we would have to bleach the hair first to remove some of the colour and create a blonde shade to which we could then add the red colour. This is one way that we can create the more avant-garde hairstyles or the really adventurous punk styles.

Colours also absorb and reflect each other. Where more than one colour is being used, take care that the colours don't clash. They must look good together.

When colour or bleach is being applied to the hair for the first time, the hair is called 'virgin hair'. This type of hair is usually the best for colouring competitions because the condition of the hair is unaffected by any previous hair-dressing process. In competitions it's usually the bright colours that win because they stand out and catch the eye of the judge.

Some styles look good with just part of the haircut coloured, the colours show off the significant lines and techniques. Good colour can make an average haircut look great.

A good hairstylist has a sound knowledge of the many types of artificial colour, as well as understanding the complementary colours, such as yellow which complements blue, and red which complements green. These colours look good together. Nature has a way of mixing the right colours together in harmony. But artificial colours can easily be applied which simply don't look right together. A good all-round knowledge means that the hairdresser will be able to do pleasant basic colour changes or the more dramatic bright colours seen in punk styles, etc.

Natural colouring is available such as henna, which is made from the leaves of an Egyptian privet plant. It has been used on hair for many years to add shine and condition as well as some lovely warm red shades. Henna was even used by the ancient Egyptians to dye their fingernails so it's difficult to remove. If you want to use it on your own hair, remember to wear gloves. Henna will go deeply into the cuticle and it could be classed as a semi-rinse. Other natural colours used to be made from nuts and blackcurrants, etc., but the artificial colours have improved so much over the years that the use of natural colouring is becoming less widespread.

If you intend to use home brands and are not sure which will dye your hair permanently, you will be able to judge this once you open the box. If it is a permanent tint it will probably contain a bottle of hydrogen peroxide which needs mixing with the colour before the tint is applied.

Remember that hydrogen peroxide is added so that the tint can go deeper into the hair; hydrogen peroxide is not just used as a lightener. A weaker percentage is needed even whilst making the hair darker when using the permanent tint.

Always read the instructions thoroughly before beginning any hairdressing procedure. Wear rubber gloves and make sure that you don't drop colour onto your skin. Wrap an old towel round your shoulders or better still put some old clothes on. You can ruin clothes by dropping colour on them. It takes a while to get the colour off your skin as well.

If you have any doubts about using any home products on certain types of hair, one way you can avoid damaging the hair is to do a test.

If the hair is to be coloured then snip a little hair off – perhaps during a haircut – and apply colour to it following the mixing instructions, just as you would if you were doing the whole style. This shows you exactly what colour you can expect from the product and how it will affect the condition of your hair.

If your whole hairstyle doesn't need cutting at the time, just cut enough hair for the test. You don't need to cut much off and if your hair is quite long you might be able to snip some off without anyone noticing that it has been cut. Cut a piece either from the back or underneath the main length of hair. Don't cut right down to the roots, but try to leave a couple of inches to blend into the style.

Highlights

Highlights make a dull-looking hairstyle and colour shade

more interesting. Hydrogen peroxide is mixed with bleach and applied to separate strands of hair. What really happens is that the process takes colour out of the hair. The knack is to stop the action at the desired shade. One method is to pick strands out and apply the mixture, then wrap in tinfoil. This method is slow, although it is regarded as one of the best.

The commonest technique is the cap method. This is known as a tip cap, made of polythene with holes all over it. Hair is drawn through the holes with a crochet hook and then the bleaching mixture is applied. Only experience will tell what strength of mixture to use for your base shade, and how long the process should take for the desired result. Usually 9% (30 vol.) hydrogen peroxide is mixed with bleach and applied over the hair that has been pulled through the holes in the cap. The hair is not pasted down onto the cap but rather left to stand out – this allows the oxygen to get to it. A plastic bag is placed over it, and then you must wait for the procedure to take effect. The lightening process can take anything from 5 to 20 minutes depending on hair type.

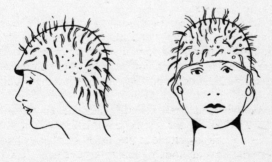

Fig. 67. Highlights.
Strands of hair pulled through a tip cap, ready for application.

If hair is very dark then you may have to use a stronger hydrogen peroxide percentage, e.g. 12% (40 vol.). If this is the case, check the hair every couple of minutes. With dark hair you may also find the lightening process takes a little longer.

Special effects

Sometimes you want to look different for just one night, perhaps a wild night out at a party, with a really unusual hairstyle, one that isn't permanent. Here are some things you can do without damaging your hair.

CRIMPING

Crimping is a good method of creating a very different hairstyle that is not permanent. Hair can be crimped to stand up and out from the head or simply all crimped down into shape. The crimping iron is a sandwich iron that creates undulations in the hair using heat. There are different sorts of crimping patterns that create wide or thin undulations.

Crimping should only be done once or twice a month. A couple of times each week would certainly damage the hair. In my opinion very fine hair should rarely (if ever) be crimped.

GEL

Setting gel can be bought in most salons and many chemists. With gel you can give a curly perm a permanent wet look, or you can dry the gel into the hair whilst styling it which will fix the hair into position. Hair can be made to stand up, or move a particular way, and will hold the style until it gets damp. Experiment until you find the effect you want.

MOUSSE

Hair mousse is ideal for giving the style more volume as well as setting it in place. It's easier and more convenient than blow-dry lotion and there are a great number of makes available. Some of them are even semi-permanent colours.

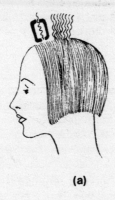

(a)

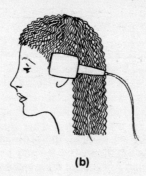

(b)

Fig. 68. Crimping.
(a) Making the hair stand up on a short layered bob.
(b) Crimping a long bob.

GLITTER SPRAYS

Sprays are also popular in bright colours, or even in silver or gold. The spray washes off easily and looks great at Christmas parties, guaranteed to turn a few heads.

BEADS

Beads are popular. They need to be firmly fixed and you may have to hunt round for some that are suitable for hair.

WIGS AND THINGS

For that special occasion, wigs may be ideal. There are many inexpensive colourful ones on the market. You may even have strangers wondering whether it is your real hair or not.

You can buy pieces of hair for pony tails and plaits which attach to your real hair. There are many other things you can add to your hair: pieces of material, feathers, colourful slides and hair grips, hair jewellery, and flowers. A colourful hat will show off the right hairstyle. People come up with new ideas all the time. A good head of hair is a thing of beauty and deserves further decoration!

HAIR'S TO THE FUTURE

New scientific breakthroughs are made every year. Hair transplants are becoming more successful. Even a cure for baldness is said to have been developed although it may be a long time before it is widely available and successful for all hair types. But I am sure that scientists will find the complete cure for baldness one day.

Hairstylists will continue to create new styles, but they won't all be new. Some will be stolen from history books, old paintings, or other cultures.

Fashion is always changing. Perhaps it is due to boredom and the desire to be different. The most unusual styles become accepted as the norm when they become fashionable. So anything is possible for future hairstyles. Maybe there will come a complete reversal of style, with more feminine styles for men, and more macho-looking ones for women. New methods of cutting will always be appearing because of the fashion movement and the creative hairstylist. Anything *can* be made fashionable. The fashion industry deliberately creates new trends so as to sell new products. With mass advertising they can promote new styles and enhance their sales.

Youngsters often adopt way-out hairstyles as part of the "uniform", sometimes doing their hair a great injustice! Hairstyles can be distinctive to the point of setting groups of people and cultures apart. Some religions adopt their own particular hairstyle to distinguish them from others and make them recognisable. All of these things remind us of the importance of hairstyle.

You can choose a style that is unique. You may even create a hairstyle yourself by taking your idea to a hairstylist. Most hairdressers enjoy experimenting and creating something new. The future will bring forth some startling changes in the world of hairdressing. I will try to keep an open mind!

8

THE HAIRDRESSING SALON

Searching for a good hairstylist

What I have said so far in this book has been aimed at helping you to style someone's hair at home. But almost no-one can rely entirely on partner, relative or friend to carry out all the jobs that are needed. There must be times when you call in the professional, the expert hairstylist, who may become your friend as well.

So in this final short chapter I give advice on choosing salon and stylist, and I make some suggestions for those who are considering a career in hairdressing.

Any small town or even village may have anything up to five hair salons. A big city may possess more than a hundred scattered around. Even a small salon may have up to five or more hairdressers. Finding the hairstylist to suit you is not always easy.

The hairdresser you choose to cut your hair may be a specialist, perhaps brilliant at cutting and blowstyling hair but not so brilliant at permanent waving. This may seem odd but there are many different arts involved in hairdressing. Sometimes stylists find that they love only one aspect of their trade and neglect the others. If they happen to own the salon, they might employ someone to perm and highlight hair whilst they do the cutting, for example. I consider this a waste of talent, but even so there are some exceptional specialist hairdressers.

Your problem is to find one stylist who can cater for your individual needs.

There are many types of hair salon even some with owners who are not involved in hairdressing at all. It is possible that someone has simply wanted to open a salon – employing hairdressers – and then decides to learn the trade from the people employed as well as by attending courses.

When you walk into a salon for the first time, remember that size doesn't always equal quality. A large salon with a lot of staff may contain some exceptional stylists, but this may be just as true of a small one.

A good salon should be smart and clean and you should be made to feel welcome. Usually the state of the salon reflects the attitude of its hairdressers. If the salon looks as if they couldn't care less, you can be sure their standard of hairdressing will be similar.

You may be visiting the salon or asking for a named stylist on a friend's recommendation. This is one of the most common forms of introduction. Be careful. Don't just rush into the salon and allow them to do anything they like to your hair. Have a good talk to the stylist. Find out the hairdresser's opinion. If it is your first visit to the salon, tread carefully. It may be wise to have a slight trim; next time you should feel more at ease having your hair styled or permed.

It's important to find out whether the hairdresser is experienced in catering for the style you want. Some stylists hate to admit they can't do something. They will always have a go and damn the consequences!

Here's an old hairdressing joke:

A man walks into a hair salon, the hairdresser greets him and asks him how he would like his hair cut.

"Cut a big chunk out of the back, chop the fringe into a lopsided cut, and shred the layers into short stumpy lumps at the sides."

"I can't do that Sir," the hairdresser answers, amazed.

"Then why did you do that the last time I was here?"

Despite this, I believe the general standard of hairdressing in this country is very good. But at the moment in Britain anyone can legally set up in business as a hairdresser – there are no laws in force to prohibit this.

There are however a number of ways for someone to become a *qualified* hairdresser.

There are private schools offering courses at various standards.

There are indentured apprenticeships offering a good practical training in hairstyling (using the teaching methods favoured by that particular salon).

There are technical college courses leading to formal qualifications; sometimes the colleges leave it to the salon to improve the practical training.

There are schemes that offer a mixture of salon training and college training.

To be honest, there are exceptional hairdressers springing from all these methods of training. It should be remembered however that the pioneers of hairdressing had no qualifications and they lived not so long ago. You may find a good salon with diplomas on the wall, but you may also find a salon with no diplomas on the wall which offers the same high standard, since many hairdressers do not display qualifications.

The only real way the general public can know what to expect from a salon is to rely on reputation, by seeing the standard of work they do at that particular salon or from knowing people who go there regularly.

Hairdressing encompasses so many skilful arts that even with diplomas there will still be things worth learning. The best hairdresser you can possibly find is one that has an open mind, and loves working with hair and who will therefore strive to give you the best possible hairstyle.

Salon equipment

HOOD DRYERS
 Used for drying sets into place, etc.

ACCELERATOR
 This has a hood as well, but it produces infra-red heat.

OCTOPUS
A group of arms that end in infra-red bulbs to dry stationary styles such as curly perms, etc.

HYDRAULIC CHAIRS
Chairs that can be raised or lowered. They make the hairdresser's job a lot easier.

STERILISER
There are many types of steriliser available to keep hairdressing tools clean.

BACKWASH AND FORWARDWASH BASINS
Hairdressing basins are a different size and shape from the usual household basin. They have been created specially for convenience in hairdressing.

DRESSING OUT AND WORK UNITS
A work unit usually has a good-sized working mirror and shelves and drawers for clippers, etc.

FIRE EXTINGUISHER
Should be found in every salon, and regularly serviced.

NORMAL TOOLS
Tongs, hairdryers, scissors, electric shears, razors. A selection of hair grips, trolleys, rollers, perm rods, combs, brushes and many more.

Working in a salon
I enjoy my work. If I'm to spend a third of my life working, I make a point of enjoying it. I make my work fun, the only difference between hard work and good fun is attitude. I search for ways to make the job more exciting and more rewarding.

I meet new people every day. The atmosphere in a good salon is very friendly. The job itself is stimulating and creative. Hairdressing is an art form, working with colour harmony, texture and shapes. A pair of scissors in the hands of a skilful hair artist does more than just cut hair, it creates new patterns. It makes asymmetrical and symmetrical shapes that are in harmony and bring out the best from human features. Hairdressing is a very personal art that must cater for each individual.

Most modern salons have music playing to relax the client and the hairstylist. I have seen many hairdressers work to music; it helps to keep their rhythm. Everything has rhythm: the music, the movement of the hairdresser, the cut and style, the click of the scissors, each breath we breathe, and even our heartbeat. A hair salon has its own rhythm, it may be very fast or very slow, depending on the trade and the people running it. In our salons we cater for all types of hairstyle and all types of person. The rhythm in our salons is fast and efficient and we train and motivate our staff to keep to that pace.

Dealing with a varied selection of people each week, I have experienced most hair problems and put the necessary solutions into effect many times. Hairstyling relates to a great many things, and to a woman and indeed a man hair is an essential part of good looks.

A well-run salon makes a client welcome from the first moment of stepping through the door. When I visit a restaurant I expect good service and feel an obligation to try to give good service in my own trade. Once the client's hair is prepared for the beginning of the hairstyling process I make absolutely sure that I know exactly what the client wants. Some clients want to be advised on a new style and others know what they want from the start. There are some salons that tend to style hair regardless of what the client has asked for. Perhaps they have come to forget that the client is the most important part of hairstyling. Without the client the business doesn't exist!

With the popularity of unisex styling, both sexes are usually quite happy having their hair styled in the same place. This gives hairdressers the perfect opportunity to develop their art and learn different aspects of hairdressing. Both our salons are unisex salons. I find it hard to understand why some hairdressers stop learning and begin to turn trade away by refusing to offer either one service or the other.

Very large salons may have hair specialists who cater for just one aspect of our art, and this is fine for the really big salon.

Colour scheme is important. Bright friendly colours are essential and they must complement each other.

People constantly ask me what sort of styling I like to do most. To be honest I have no particular favourites. No doubt if I was just doing one style over and over again I would soon be bored. In a busy working day a booking column may be full of a selection of cuts and perms, highlights, colours and sets. The wider the variety, the more interesting it is.

Every year we have to improve our shops or our skills in some way. Sometimes a business seems like a monster that must constantly be fed. The larger it gets the more food it needs. To make the business larger, one must make the workload larger. Often for a business to survive it has to expand, to compete with the other businesses around it.

Some salons get up to all sorts of tricks to improve their trade; poaching staff is one of them. A hairdresser soon builds up a clientele by working in a salon for a number of years. If the stylist leaves, the clientele will often follow, taking trade from one salon to another, or to a new salon if he sets up in business on his own.

Sometimes salons get a member of staff to 'phone their rivals enquiring about prices, pretending to be a possible client. They then try to compete by reducing their own prices to a slightly lower figure. But equally one can compete by offering better quality and service. I would rather offer an honest service for an honest price.

So you want to be a hairdresser?

How does the young person enter the world of hairdressing?

The first obvious way is to become an indentured apprentice, or to opt for the Youth Training Scheme. A salon that takes apprentices may have its own training facilities, or may send apprentices to day-release courses at college. Each salon has different styles and ideas of training.

Another way is to start a full-time hairdressing course at

technical college. Once you are qualified, a salon should employ you as an improver. The work within a salon differs from that involved at college. An improver will begin practical hairdressing in the salon, under supervision for the remainder of the qualification period.

In any case, if you want to start learning about hairdressing, you should start a Saturday job, perhaps before leaving school. You can then learn the day-to-day techniques involved. It would enable a potential employer to see how keen you are, and help you to decide whether hairdressing is really the career for you. Hairdressing isn't as glamorous as some people imagine, it can be very hard work!

Some salons have their own training schools. They offer all sorts of styling tuition and hairdressing refresher courses, most of which have some kind of diploma at the end of them. Sometimes they are expensive but they are often very good for cramming knowledge into you as well as letting you practise the mechanics of hairdressing in intensive training. Potential employers may be impressed by a trainee with advance cutting diplomas.

It's never too late to learn hairdressing. Technical colleges or private schools are usually available for anyone. I have known some people make a career-change or simply go along to courses because they are interested in styling. Hairdressing offers many prospects. You may become self-employed. You may work on board a liner that cruises around the world. You may decide to teach hairdressing or simply enjoy working in a hair salon designing hairstyles and perhaps creating new ones.

Starting a hairdressing business

Hairdressing businesses range from the door-to-door hairdresser to the small salon owner, and on to the large chains of salons.

Before you open your first salon, check these points:

Is it the right place? Location is vital – on it may depend success or failure. Consider the amount of trade and the amount of competition. Create your salon environment to suit the type of trade you intend to cater for.

Some salons prosper even in less promising places by building up a good reputation. They must try harder to build their business because they have to attract people to travel further to their salon.

Some small village salons may do better than large city ones because of lower rent and rates.

If you want a small salon, it might be wise to buy rather than rent if you can find a mortgage for more or less the same outgoings.

People are naturally cautious when starting a business, but there should be no half measures. It's no good being obsessed by the possibility of failure.

The best way to build a business is to offer a first-class service at a reasonable price. If your price is too high you will price yourself out of the market. If your price is too low people will think that your hairdressing is second-rate. Once you start to style people's hair well, you will be surprised at how quickly the news spreads!

How can you advertise? Use hair shows, demonstrations, and fashion shows incorporating your hairstyles. Promotion such as T shirts, hats or beer mats with your salon logo printed on. Competitions run by your salon in local newspapers and magazines. Normal adverts on radio. Posters, leaflets, donations of half-price styling to local organisations, and many more.

You must find out what works best for your salon; all salons are different. It may pay simply to concentrate on your local trade, building a reputation and eventually it will spread, people will come looking for you.

What about overheads? Wages, telephones, electricity, insurance, rates and rent or mortgage. Tax, VAT, stock purchase, staff, advertising, accountant, possible bank loan, solicitor, and many others. The list is daunting, and people don't know where to start.

The best thing is to estimate all your expenses, add what you need to live on yourself, and then work out what turnover your salon must make to survive. Profit can be increased by cost-effective advertising, acceptable price increases, cutting down on unnecessary spending, adding new lines of sale, and of course good quality work, good salesmanship, and excellent reputation.

STAFF

Choosing the right people is essential but difficult. Some people are time-wasters or have the wrong attitude, or lack experience. The staff you choose will make or break your salon. Attitude is important. They need a pleasant manner, complemented by a genuine desire to work and style hair to the best of their ability. The staff must work well together, helping each other through the busy times.

It is important that they don't feel that they know everything. One question I sometimes ask at interviews is "How do you cope with mistakes". One hairdresser answered, "I never make mistakes". This attitude doesn't work. Human beings all make mistakes. We want confident people who will cope with many types of hairdressing, but the list of hairdressing skills is so vast that no hairdresser can be an expert at everything.

If you set up in business, be prepared for hard work. It is a misconception that the businessman sits back and reaps the rewards whilst his staff do all the work. There are hundreds of things to do and at least one seemingly major problem each week. If you own a lock-up shop you may be awoken at 3 a.m. to be told your shop has been broken into, or your display window has been smashed.

If you are determined to go into business, none of these things will put you off. Have a balanced attitude towards problems. There will always be more people ready to talk you out of it than give encouragement. It's no use being frightened of failure and it's only yourself that you are failing if you don't follow your dreams. Running a business, you shape your own destiny. One day you will look back with pride at the things you have achieved.

For great hair you need

A PERFECT CUT

The haircut is the foundation of the hairstyle. Without

proper cutting, the style will look second-rate.

GOOD CONDITION

Condition affects everything we do to hair. With poor condition, perms and other methods of styling never look good.

HEALTH

Keep fit, keep yourself healthy, it will show in your hair.

HAIRSTYLIST

Visit a good hairstylist who will solve all your hair problems given time. The stylist will choose an individual style for you, perhaps adding complementary colours to enhance the style, and perms to give movement.

9

CONCLUSION

I can't stress enough how important even a little knowledge of your hair is. A head of hair should be treated with the same respect you might give to a very expensive mink coat, and yet hair as a natural and beautiful fashion asset is very often taken for granted.

The mink coat will be worn occasionally but your hair will be with you every minute of the day. It is always there being judged by those who see you and it may at times even give an insight into your personality.

Wild flowing hair would seem to denote an exciting individual making that person seem much more interesting. Hair can be styled to emphasise the best points of your features making the most of what you've got. It can make you look drab and boring or make you seem to radiate confidence.

We can't always hurry to a hair salon to keep our hair looking good, so there will always be times when the ability to style your own hair will be invaluable.

If you've read through the book I hope you've enjoyed it and I am sure that with a little practice you will become very competent at Hairstyling At Home.

BEST WISHES
RICHARD GILROY

Index

OUR PUBLISHING POLICY

HOW WE CHOOSE

Our policy is to consider every deserving manuscript and we can give special editorial help where an author is an authority on his subject but an inexperienced writer. We are rigorously selective in the choice of books we publish. We set the highest standards of editorial quality and accuracy. This means that a *Paperfront* is easy to understand and delightful to read. Where illustrations are necessary to convey points of detail, these are drawn up by a subject specialist artist from our panel.

HOW WE KEEP PRICES LOW

We aim for the big seller. This enables us to order enormous print runs and achieve the lowest price for you. Unfortunately, this means that you will not find in the *Paperfront* list any titles on obscure subjects of minority interest only. These could not be printed in large enough quantities to be sold for the low price at which we offer this series.

   We sell almost all our *Paperfronts* at the same unit price. This saves a lot of fiddling about in our clerical departments and helps us to give you world-beating value. Under this system, the longer titles are offered at a price which we believe to be unmatched by any publisher in the world.

OUR DISTRIBUTION SYSTEM

Because of the competitive price, and the rapid turnover, *Paperfronts* are possibly the most profitable line a bookseller can handle. They are stocked by the best bookshops all over the world. It may be that your bookseller has run out of stock of a particular title. If so, he can order more from us at any time – we have a fine reputation for "same day" despatch, and we supply any order, however small (even a single copy), to any bookseller, as this reminds him of the strong underlying public demand for *Paperfronts*. Members of the public who live in remote places, or who are housebound, or whose local bookseller is unco-operative, can order direct from us by post.

FREE

If you would like an up-to-date list of all Paperfront titles currently available, send a stamped self-addressed envelope to
ELLIOT RIGHT WAY BOOKS, BRIGHTON RD.,
LOWER KINGSWOOD, SURREY, U.K.